BDS & CBS India
Exam. Oriented Series

ORAL HISTOLOGY AND ANATOMY

(Questions & Answers)

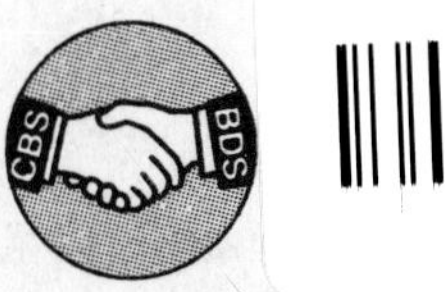

Praveen Bansal

Foreword by
Dr. Ashok Dhoble

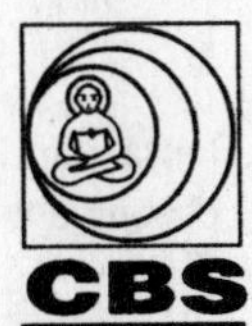

CBS PUBLISHERS & DISTRIBUTORS
NEW DELHI • BANGALORE (INDIA)

ISBN : 81-239-1460-1

First Edition : 2007
Reprint : 2009

Publishing Director : Vinod K. Jain

Published by :
Satish Kumar Jain for CBS Publishers & Distributors,
4596/1-A, 11 Darya Ganj, New Delhi - 110 002 (India)
E-mail: cbspubs@vsnl.com • Website: www.cbspd.com

Branch Office :
2975, 17th Cross, K.R. Road, Bansankari 2nd Stage, Bangalore-70
Fax : 080-26771680 • E-mail : cbsbng@vsnl.net

Composed by :
LineArt Graphics, Delhi-110091

Printed at :
Asia Printograph, Delhi

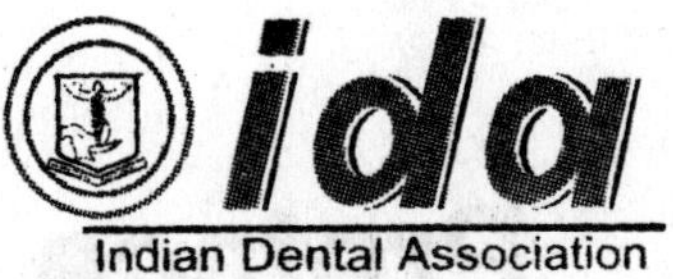

Dr. ASHOK DHOBLE
Hon. Secretary General
Bombay Mutual Terrace, 2nd Floor,
534, Sandhurst Bridge, Opera House,
Mumbai 400 007
Tel: 91-22-2364-3344/2363 6655
ashokdhoble@ida.org.in

Foreword

It gives me immense pleasure in presenting this series on Short Notes and Long Question Answer in Dentistry. The students of dental sciences face a difficult situation as they need to study their theory clubbed with clinicals and practicals. At the end of the year, although they may be good in their knowledge of theory and clinical skills, they still get tensed up due to lack of orientation towards university exam and the question paper pattern. This series has been designed specifically for this situation and I am sure it will go a long way helping the students in this direction.

Dr. Praveen Bansal is the brain behind this huge project and he took ideas and views from knowledgeable and experienced teachers, to write this series. The presentation style is catchy. I wish him all the best in this project as well as in his many more forthcoming projects.

Dr. ASHOK DHOBLE
Hon. Secretary General
Indian Dental Association, Head Office

Preface

BDS & CBS India Exam. Oriented Series is designed as pattern of long question answers, short question answers and clinical problems. The students are expected to know all the topic as well as specific information and last minute relevant details having clinical importance.

This series is structured to cover the essential aspects of BDS syllabus for quick reference in question answers format. I have tried my best to include almost all the topics presented in the syllabus by Dental Council of India in a simple language.

PRAVEEN BANSAL

Contents

Section–1

ORAL HISTOLOGY

Section–2

DENTAL ANATOMY

Section–1

ORAL HISTOLOGY

1 Development of Face and Oral Cavity

L.Q.A.1 Describe development of palate

Ans. Development of face begins at the age of 4th week of intra uterine life and at the same time that is around 28th day or 4th week, palate begins to develop (i.e. initially primary palate) and later around the 7th week the secondary palate begins to develop.

PALATE

Development begins at 4th week and completes around 9th week of intrauterine (iu) life.

Structures taking part in palate formation

Medial nasal process : Give rise to premaxillary/primary palate

Maxillary process : Give rise to secondary palate

Formation of primary palate

Initially in the 4th week after when the MNP forms, from its posterior aspect i.e. behind the middle part the lip, it forms (MNP medial nasal process) the primary palate. During this phase the M.P. (maxillary processes) continue to grow medially. In anterior region it fuses with MNP to give rise to upper lip. Posteriorly it remains unfused due to the interference of tongue.

Formation of secondary palate

Initially, the oral cavity and nasal cavity is common, and is occupied by the developing tongue, later on after the development of the palate both nasal cavity and oral cavity becomes separated.

The posterior region of maxillary process continue to grow medially and in downward direction on either side of tongue. These two process on either side of tongue are called "palatine process or shelves". This occurs at around 6th week.

After the 7th week, by the unfolding of head the tongue is withdrawn between the two palatine shelves, and provide space to palatine shelves to approximate each other. Palatine shelves now elevate and fused to primary palate as well as themselves.

Factors responsible for closer of secondary palate

(i) Unfolding of head

(ii) High glycosaminoglycan content of shelves attracts water and makes the shelves turgid

(iii) Presence of contractile fibroblast in the palatine shelves.

Fusion

By 8th to 9th week fusion occurs between the nasal septa coming from upward primary palate, and two palatine shelves.

As the palatal shelves approximates epithelial covering on each shelves adheres with each other and becomes indistinguishable. The surface epithelial cells sloughed off by physiologic cell death and basal cells get exposed. A midline seam developed which consists of two layer of basal cells. This midline seam first thins to a single layer and ultimately losts resulting into continuation of mesenchymal tissue.

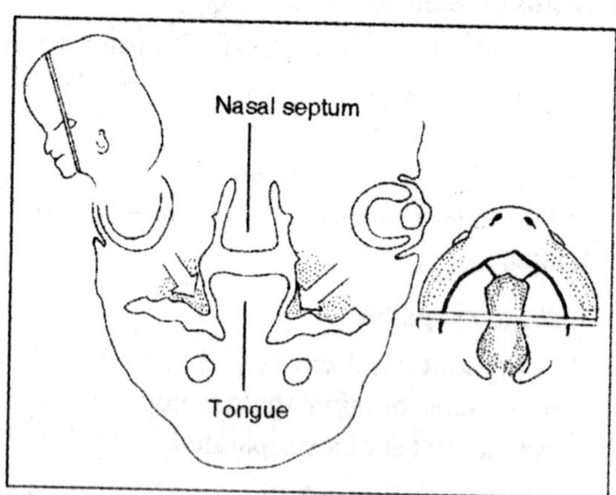

Fig- 1.1(a) At 7 weeks the palatal shelves are forming from the maxillary processes and are directed downward on either side of the developing tongue.

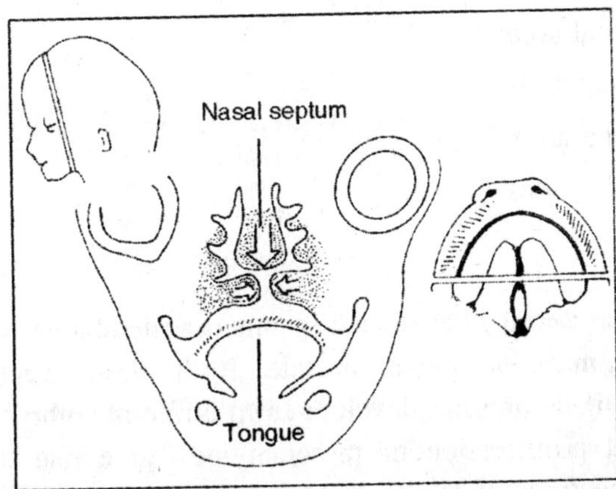

Fig- 1.1 (b) At 8 weeks the tongue has been depressed and the palatal shelves have elevated but not fused.

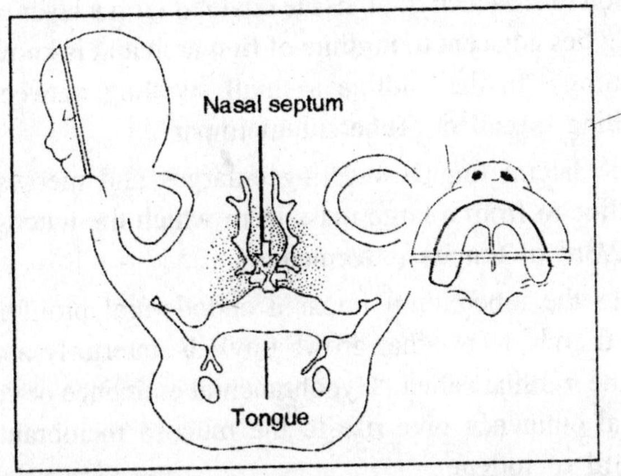

Fig- 1.1(c) Fusion of the shelves and the nasal septum is completed.

Ossification of palate

It occurs from 8th week of I.U. This is an intramembrenous type of ossification. The most posterior part of palate does not ossify, it forms soft palate. Mid palatal suture ossifies by 12-14 yrs.

S.Q.A.1 Development of tongue

Ans. Development of tongue begins at around 4th week of I.U life.

Contributing structures

- 1st brachial arch

2nd brachial arch

3rd brachial arch

4th brachial arch

Occipital somites

Development

Initially tongue develops as a sack of mucosa membrane which later on filled with a mass of lingual muscle. Both these structures, lingual mucosa and lingual muscles develops from different embryonic structure. Initially, local proliferation of mesenchyme give rise to number of swelling in the floor of the mouth from different pharyngeal arches.

At 4th week localized swelling occur in the 1st branchial arch due to proliferation of mesenchymal tissue covered with a layer of epithelium. This swelling lies adjacent to midline of first arch and is known as "lateral lingual swelling". In the midline a small swelling between the lateral lingual swelling is called "Tuberculum impar".

Later, the lateral lingual swelling enlarges and merges with each other at midline to from a large mass from which the mucosa membrane of anterior 2/3rd of tongue is formed.

Caudal to the tuberculum impar a endodermal proliferation in the middle of 3rd arch occurs that grows towards anteriorly and covers the 2nd arch in the midline called "Hypohranchial eminence or copula". This hypobranchial eminence give rise to the mucosa membrane of root, or posterior 1/3rd of tongue.

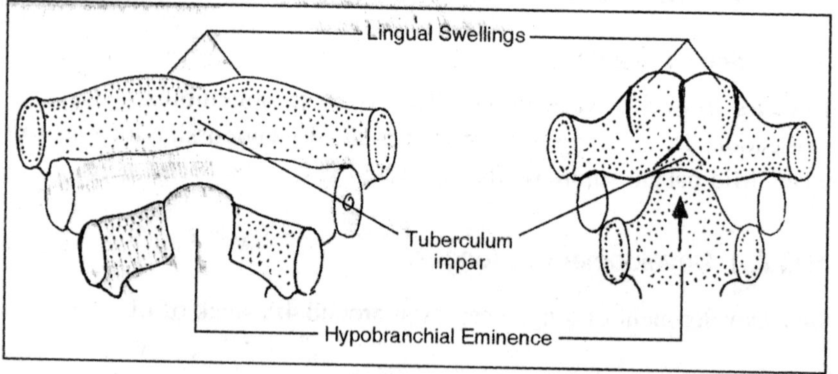

Fig. 1.2

The point at which the 1st and 2nd bronchial arches merges is marked as foramen ceacum just behind the sulcus terminalis. The tongue separates from the floor of mouth by downward growth of ectoderm around its periphery.

The muscles of tongue originates from the occipital somites which have migrated forward in to the tongue area.

S.Q.A.2 Meckels cartilage

Ans. It is a primary cartilage of 1st branchial arch (mandibular arch) It has no direct contribution in the development of mandible but it provides framework for the development of mandible. It extends from the cartilaginous otic capsule to midline or symphysis. Ossification begins at the lateral aspect of the meckels cartilage for the development of mandible and that spread along the inferior alveolar nerve around it.

A major portion of meckels cartilage disappears during growth and remaining part develops into the following structures.

- Mental ossicles
- Incus and malleus
- Spine of sphenoid bone
- Anterior ligament of malleus
- Sphenomandibular ligament
- Sphenomalleolar ligament

NOTES

2 Development and Growth of Teeth

L.Q.A.1 Describe in detail about stages of tooth development.

Ans. The embryonic oral cavity is lined by stratified squamous epithelium known as the oral ectoderm. At around 6th week of I.U the infero-lateral border of the maxillary arch and the supero-lateral border of the mandibular arch show localized proliferation of the oral ectoderm resulting in horse shoe shaped band of tissue called "Dental lamina". The ectoderm in certain areas of the dental lamina proliferates and forms a knob like structures that grow into underlying mesenchyma. Each of these knob are called "Enamel organ". As the development progresses it increases in size and changes in shape. Depending upon the shape of enamel organ, it is dividing into following stages.

- Bud stage
- Cap stage
- Bell stage
- Advance bell stage

These stages are also called " Morphologic stages".

BUD STAGE

This is the initial stage of enamel organ represented by 1st epithelial inclusion into the ectomesenchyme.

Histologically the stage have low coloumnar cells peripherally and polygonal cells centrally. The surrounding mesenchyme undergo mitosis. As a result of the increased mitotic activity and migration of neural crest cells in to the area, results in condensation of ectomenchyme in two areas.

The area of condensation just below the enamel organ is the " Dental papilla" later which give rise to dental pulp and dentin. The area of condensation that surrounds the enamel organ is called "Dental sac" which in future give rise to part of periodontium [cementum and PDL]

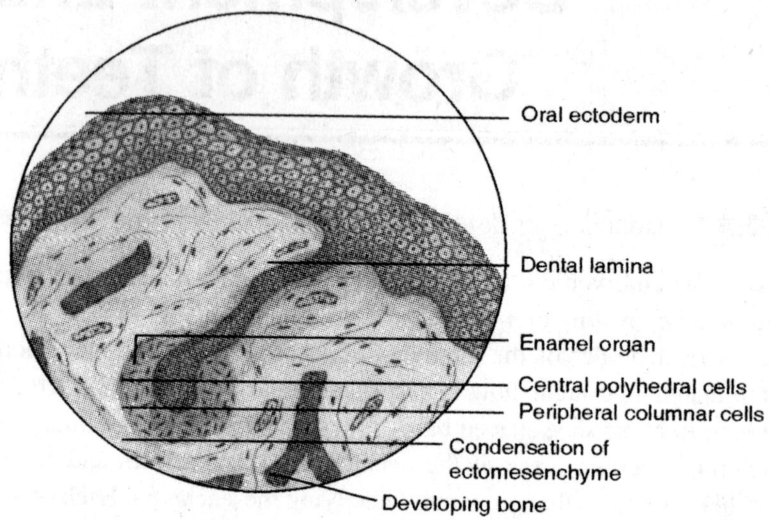

Fig. 2.1: Bud stage of tooth development (Ref. Fig. 3.1–Maji jose)

CAP STAGE

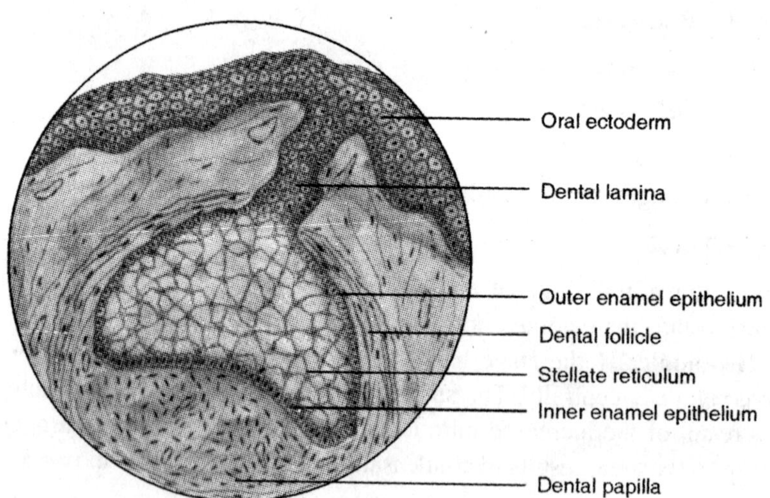

Fig. 2.2: Cap stage of tooth development (Ref. Fig. 3.2–Maji jose)

As the bud stage continues to proliferate it does not expand uniformly through out. It proliferate unequally giving rise to cap stage characterized by a shallow invagination.

Histology

Outer and inner enamel epithelium: Cells that covering the convexity of the enamel organ at this stage are called outer enamel epithelium. These cells are cuboidal cells. The tall columnar cells lining the concavity of the cap are called or referred as inner enamel epithelium.

Both the inner enamel epithelium and outer enamel epithelium are separated from dental papilla and dental sac respectively by a delicate basement meurbrane.

Stellate reticulum [Enamel pulp]: These are polygonal cell located between the inner and outer enamel epithelium, acquire more intercellular fluid and forms a cellular network called the stellate reticulum.

Dental papilla: During this stage the dental papilla further proliferate condenses and becomes more pronounced than earlier stages

Dental sac: Marginal condensation is the ectomesenchyme surrounding the enamel organ and dental papilla, gradually a more denser and fibrous layer develops. This results in primitive dental sac.

BELL STAGE

As the proliferation and invagination of epithelium continues the enamel organ assumes bell stage

Histology

On histological examination of bell stage four different types of cells are distinguished.

Inner enamel epithelium: Single layer of cells that differentiate prior to amelogenesis into tall columnar cells called "Ameloblast". These cells are attached each other by junctional complex laterally and to stratum intermedium by desmosomes. The inner enamel epithelium exert an influence on underlying mesenchymal cell which later differentiate into Odonoblasts.

Stratum intermedium: Few layer of squamous cells appears between inner enamel epithelium and stellate reticulum. These cells shows high degree of metabolic activity and this layer seems to be essential for enamel formation. This layer is absent in root portion.

Satellite reticulum: Star shaped cells present in between stratum intermedium and outer enamel epithelium. This layer further expand due to continued accumulation of intra- cellular fluid. As the enamel formation begins this layer begins to collapse to a narrow zone

Outerenamel epithelium: The cells that covers the outer periphery of the enamel organ are flattened to form low cuboidal cells. The outer enamel epithelium have fold between which adjacent mesenchyme carrying capillary loops are present which provide nutrition to the enamel orgam. A junction where inner enamel epithelium and outer enamel epithelium meets is called "Cervical loop"

Dental papilla: Dental papilla is enclosed in the invaginated portion of the enamel organ under the influence of inner enamel epithelium the peripheral cells of mesenchymal tissue differentiated into Odontoblast

The basement membrane that separates the enamel organ and dental papilla prior to the dentin formation is called "Membrana preformative" later which persist as DEJ.

Dental sac: Dental sac shows a circular arrangement of its fibres and resembles a capsular structure. As root develops, these fibres differentiate into periodontal fibres.

ADVANCE BELL STAGE

The junction between inner enamel epithelium and odontoblasts outlines the future DEJ and the cervical portion (i.e. cervical loop) give rise to Hertwig's root sheath.

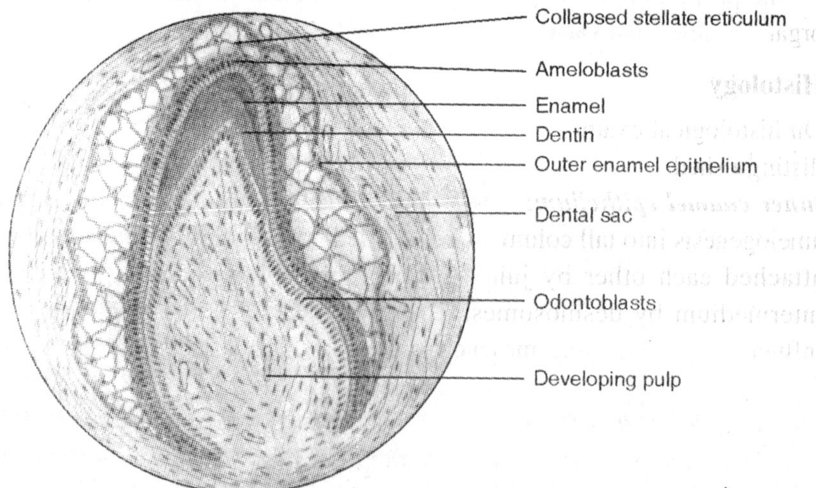

Fig. 2.3: Advanced bell stage of tooth development (Ref. Fig. 3.4–Maji jose)

During the advance bell stage following structure appears in the enamel orgam

- Inner enamel epithelium
- Stratum inter medium
- Stellate reticulum
- Outer enamel epithelium
- Cervical loop
- Dental papilla
- Dental sac

L.Q.A.2 Describe development of roots

Ans. Once the enamel and dentin formation reaches to the future CEJ the cervical loop further grow and root formation begins. The cervical loop give rise to the Hertwig's root sheath. Hertwig's root sheath consist of inner and outer enamel epithelium. Inner enamel epithelium continues to induce the proliferation of odontoblast and the 1st layer of dentin is laid down. After that if looses its structural continuity and exposing the dental follicle to dentin and the remnant of sheath present in periodontal ligament as rests cells of malassez. Dental follicle under the influence of dentin, prolifrates to form cementoblast and cementum is deposited; in this way single rooted tooth is formed.

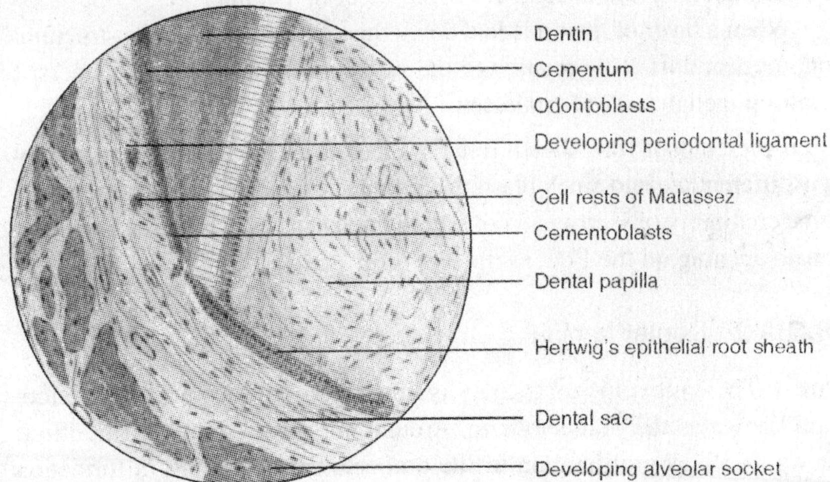

Fig. 2.4: Development of root (Ref. Fig. 3.5–Maji jose)

But in cases of multirooted teeth the root sheath produces tongue like projection of epithelium toward each other. Two tongue forms two apical foramina and three tongue forms three apical foramina converting the primary apical foramina These tongues are also called diaphragm.

The proliferation of the cells of the epithelial diaphragm is accompanied by proliferation of the cells of connnective tissue of pulp. The differentiation of odontoblasts and the formation of dentin follow the lengthening of the root sheath At the same time the connective tissue of dental sac surrounding the root sheath proliferates and invades the continuous double epithelial layer. Differential growth of the epithelial diaphragm in multirooted teeth causes the division of the root trunk into two or three roots

S.Q.A.1 Write briefly about Hertwig's root sheath

Ans. As enamel organ further develops the root begins to develop only after the enamel and dentin formation has been reached to future CEJ The root formation begins with formation of Hertwig's root sheath. Hertwig's root sheath is a continuation of cervical loop that consist of outer and inner enamel epithelium. This play an important role in the formation of root. This sheath of epithelial cells grows around the dental papilla between the papilla and follicle until it encloses all but the basal portion of the papilla. The rim of this root sheath, the epithelial diaphragm encloses the primary apical foramen. The inner cells they influences and initiate the differentiation of odonoblast from the cells of papilla.

When a layer of dentin is laid down this root sheath loses its structural continuity and its close relation to the surface of root. Its remnants persist as an epithelial rests of malassez.

If the cells of root sheath remain adherent to the dentin surface they may differentiate into ameloblasts and produce enamel, called enamel pearl" If the continuity of Hertwigs root sheath breaks, it results in accessory root canals opening on the PDL surface of root.

S.Q.A.2 Dental lamina

Ans. The embryonic oral cavity is lined by stratified squamous epithelium known as the oral ectoderm. Around 6th week of intra utrine life it shows localized proliferation of the oral ectoderm resulting in formation of horse shoe shaped band of tissue called the Dental lamina.

Dental lamina plays an important role in development of dentition. Deciduous teeth are formed directly from dental lamina permanent molars as a result of distal extension while permanent teeth that replace the deciduous teeth from the lingual extension of dental lamina.

Total activity of dental lamina is extended over a period of 5 yrs. However the dental lamina may still be active in the 3rd molar region even though it has disappeared in other area.

S.Q.A.3 Bell stage of tooth development

Ans. This stage is described on the basis of its shape (Morphological stage) that assumes a bell.

On histologic examination four types of cells are distinguished in enamel organ

- *Outer enamel epithelium:* Covers outer periphery and are flattened to form low cuboidal cells.
- *Stellate reticulum:* Star shaped cell lies between the outer enamel epithelium and stratum intermedium
- *Stratum intermedium:* Few layers of squamous cells lies between stellate reticulum & inner enamel epithelium. These cells shows high degree of metabolic activity.
- *Inner enamel epithelium:* Single layer of cells that differentiate prior to amelogenesis into tall columnar cells called ameloblast. Under the influence of inner enamel epithelium the dental papilla differentiate into odonoblast

Dantal papilla

It is enclosed in the invaginated portion of enamel organ which in future give rise to dental pulp and dentin.

Dantal sac

Connective tissue structure that surrounds the enamel organ are in future give rise to periodontal ligament and cementum

S.Q.A.4 Write the layers of Hertwig's epithelial root sheath and its role in tooth development

Ans. Two layers of Hertwig's root sheath

- Inner enamel epithelium
- Outer enamel epithelium

It has important role in the formation of root. Once the enamel and dentin formation reaches to future CEJ, root formation begins. The hertwigs root sheath grows around the dental papilla apically and the inner cell layer influences the cell of papilla to differentiate into odontoblast and 1st layer of dentin is laid down.

After the dentin is laid down the Hertwig's sheath fragment there by making the surrounding connective tissue to come in contact with dentin and proliferates into cementoblast. In case of multirooted teeth prior to root formation begins, it bends to form diaphragm which helps in the formation of multiple roots.

S.Q.A.5 Dental sac

Ans. It is a ectomesenchymal tissue that condensed around the enamel organ from the beginning of the bud stage to bell stage. This ectomesenchyme tissue becomes denser and denser and more fibrous, ultimately forming periodontal ligament and cementum.

S.Q.A.6 Histophysiological stages of tooth development.

Ans. Histophysiological stages

- Initiation
- Proliferation
- Histodiffereutiation
- Morphodifferentiation
- Apposition

Except the stage of initiation all other stages overlap and many are continues throughout various morphologic stages of odontogenesis.

S.Q.A.7 Vestibular lamina

Ans. In each dental arch labial and buccal to the dental lamina an epithelial thickening occurs independently. This epithelial thickening is called vestibul lamina or lip furrow band. It subsequently hollows and forms the oral vestibule between the alveolar process and lips/ cheeks.

S.Q.A.8 Stratum intermedium

Ans. It is formed by a few layers of squamous cells that appears in the bell stage and lies between the stellate reticulum and inner enamel epithelium. These cells are attached by gap junction and desmosomes. These cells show high degree of metabolic activity and it is essential for enamel formation.

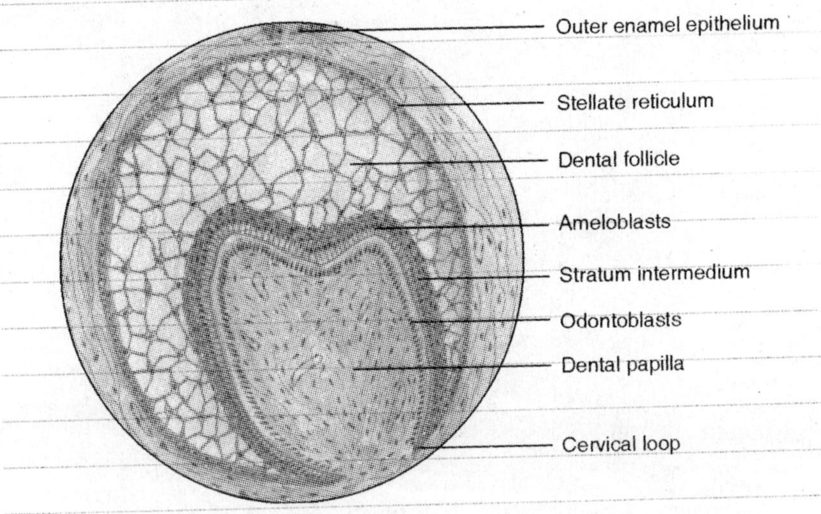

Fig. 2.5: Early bell stage of tooth development (Ref. Fig. 3.3–Maji jose)

NOTES

3

Enamel

L.Q.A.1 Describe in detail structure of enamel

Ans. Enamel is the most highly mineralized tissue consisting of 90% mineral and 4% organic material

STRUCTURE OF ENAMEL

Enamel Rods

It is a basic structural unit of enamel with a highly organized pattern of crystal orientation (hydroxyapatite crystals)

Shape: Cylindrical and is made up of crystals with their long axis running for the most part parallel to longitudinal axis of the rod

Diameter: Average of around 4μm, it varies from inner surface to outer surface The diameter of rod increases from DEJ torwards the surface at a ratio of 1:2

Course: From DEJ the rods have somewhat tortuous courses torwards surface

Length: Length is greater than the thickness of enamel because of oblique direction and wavy course

Direction of rods

Rods are oriented at right angle to the dentin surface. In cervical and central part of deciduous tooth they are horizontal. Near the incisal edge or tip of the cusps they change gradually and becomes oblique direction until they are almost verticle. Arrangement of rods in permanent teeth is same in occlusal 2/3rd but in cervical region it deviate from horizontal in an apical direction. At the cuspal or incisal edges the rod arrangement are further complicated. It seem to be interwine more irregularly This optical appearance of enamel is called Gnarled enamel

Submicroscopic structure of rods

More common pattern of prism arrangement is keyhole or paddle shaped. Rods are separated by interod substance There rods measure in 5 μm in breadth and 9 μm in length.

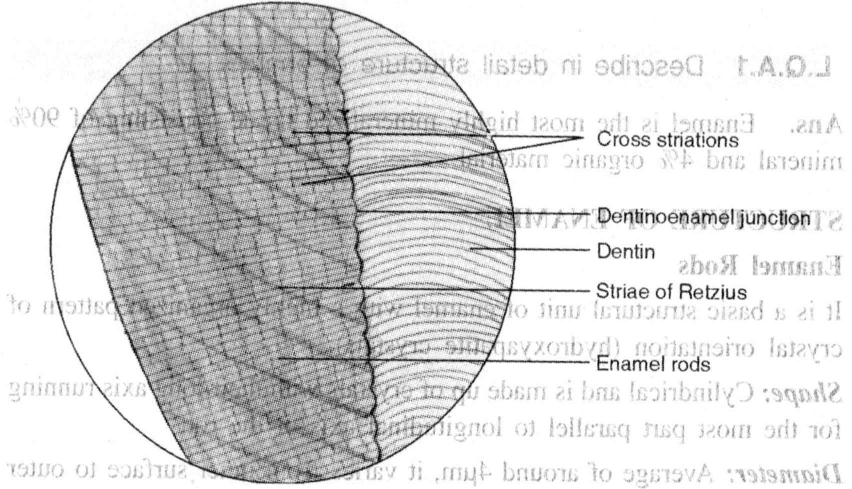

Fig. 3.1: Enamel rods – Longitudinal section (Ref. Fig. 4.1–Maji jose)

Striations

Enamel is form at a rate of approximately 4 μm per day. This results in periodic bands or cross striations. It is also reveals that there is an alternate constrictions and expansion of rods in some region resulting for this bands (scanning electron microscopy). This appearance, may also result from structural interrelations among groups of rods rather than modifications of single rod.

Bands of Hunter schreger

It is a optical phenomenon produced by changes in rod direction seen is longitudinal ground section Appears as alternating dark and light strips of varying widths. It is regarded as functional adaptation minimizing the rise of cleavage in axial direction. They starts form DEJ and ends at some distance away from surface.

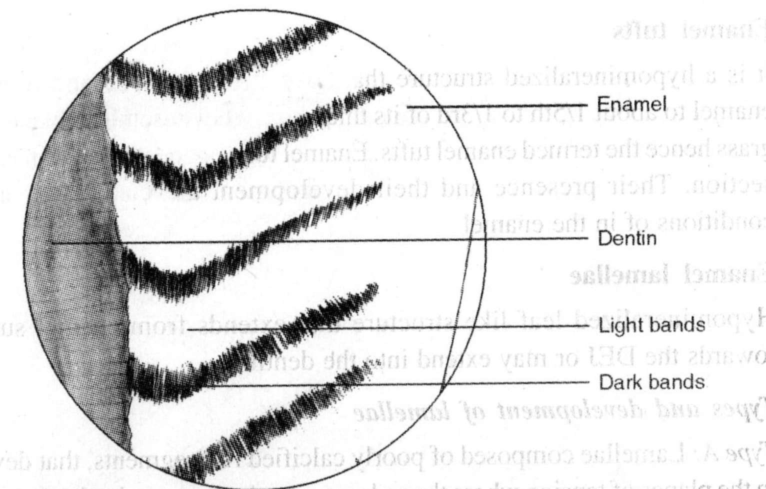

Fig. 3.2: Hunter – Schreger bands (Ref. Fig. 4.7–Maji jose)

Incremental lines of Retzius

(striae of Retzius) In ground section they appears series of dark band illustrating the incremental pattern or successive apposition of enamel during its formation. In cross section they appears as concentric circles.

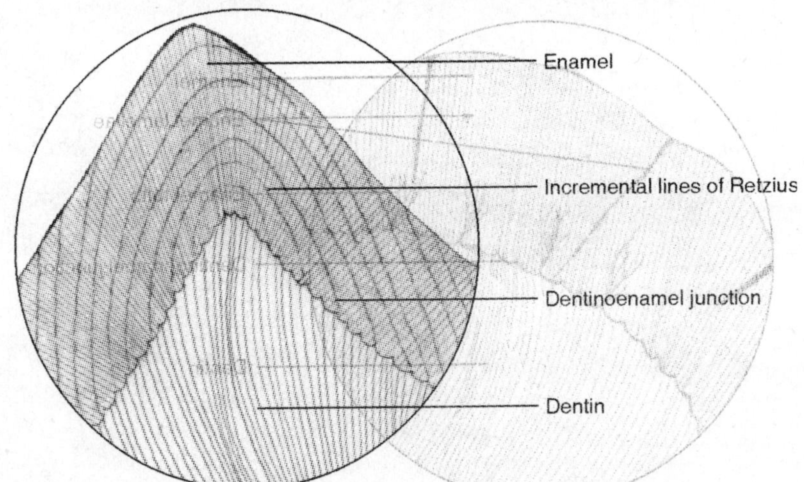

Fig. 3.3: Striae of Retzius (Ref. Fig. 4.3–Maji jose)

The exact nature of its development is not known but it have been attribute to periodic bending of enamel rods, to variation in basic organic structure or to physiologic calcification rhythm.

Enamel tufts

It is a hypomineralized structure that arises from the DEJ and runs into enamel to about 1/5th to 1/3rd of its thickness. They resembles like tufts of grass hence the termed enamel tufts. Enamel tufts are best viewed in ground section. Their presence and their development are conquence spatial conditions of in the enamel

Enamel lamellae

Hypomineralized leaf like structure that extends from enamel surface towards the DEJ or may extend into the dentin.

Types and development of lamellae

Type A: Lamellae composed of poorly calcified rod segments, that develop in the planes of tension where the rods cross such planes and a short segment of rod fails to calcify.

Type B: Lamellae consisting of degenerated cells. If the disturbance is more severe crack may result that fill with surrounding cells. This occurs when crack appears in unerupted tooth.

Type C: Lamella filled with organic material. If crack appears after eruption of tooth it is filled with surrounding organic material.

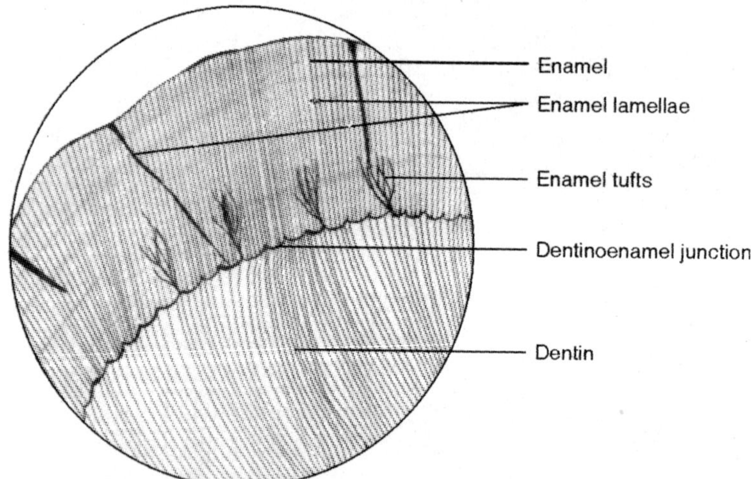

Fig. 3.4: Enamel lamellae & Enamel tufts (Ref. Fig. 4.5–Maji jose)

Enamel spindle: Occasionally odontoblastic process passes across the DEJ into the enamel thay have been term enamel spindles. It originates from odontoblastic process that extends into the enamel epithelium before hard substance are formed. Direction of enamel spindles corresponds to the original direction of ameloblasls, i.e. at right angle to dentin.

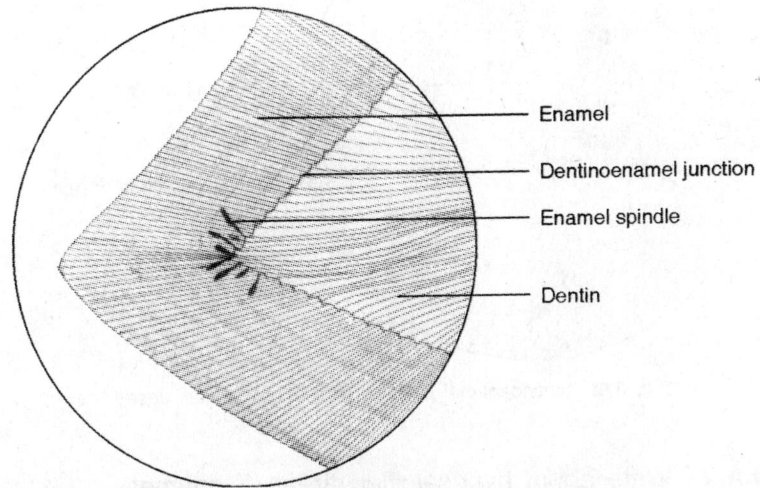

Fig. 3.5: Enamel spindles (Ref. Fig. 4.6–Maji Jose)

SURFACE STRUCTURES

The surface of enamel is characterized by several formations. The striae of Retzius often extend from DEJ to outer surface of enamel, when they end in shallow furrows known as "Perikymata". They are continuous around a tooth and usually lie parallel to each other and to CEJ.

Rod ends: Rod ends are concave and vary in depth and shape Shallowest in cervical regions of surface and deepest near incisal or occlusal surface.

Craks: Narrow fissure like structures that are seen on almost all surfaces. They are the outer edges of lamellae.

Enamel cuticle: A thin delicate membrane that covers the entire crown of newly erupted tooth but is soon removed by mastication. It is also called "Nasmyth's membrane"/primary enamel cuticle. It is typical basal lamina secreted by the ameloblasts when enamel formation is completed.

DEJ: It is a junction between dentin and enamel, establish as these two hard tissue begins to form. It has scalloped profile with convexities directed toward the dentin. The dentin surface is pitted in which rounded projections of enamel fits.

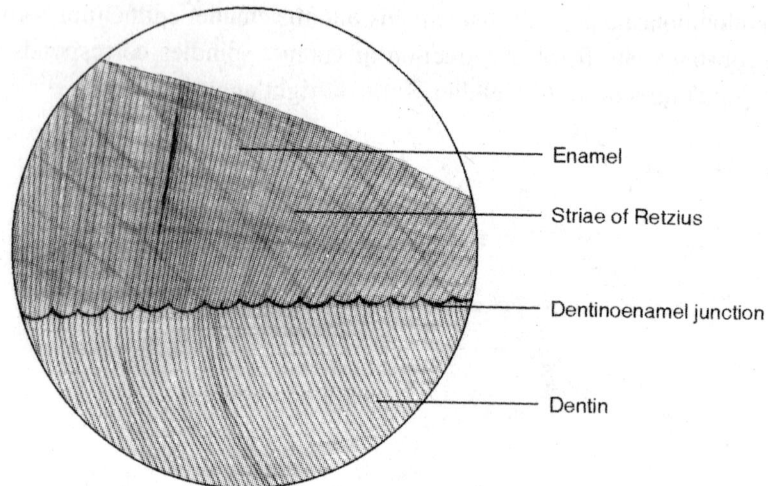

Fig. 3.6: Dentinoenamel junction (Ref. Fig. 5.4–Maji Jose)

L.Q.A.2 Write about hypocalcified areas & enamel

Ans. Following are the hypocalcified areas of enamel.

- Enamel lamellae
- Enamel tufts
- Enamel spindles
- Enamel article

Enamel lamallae

These are thin leaf like structures that extends from the enamel surface to the DEJ and some times may extends into the dentin. They consist of organic material with little mineral contents. In ground section these structure may confused with cracks.

Types of enamel lamellae and their development

Types A: Lamellae composed of poorly calcified rod segments. It develops in the plane of tension where the rods cross such plane and short segments of rods fails to calcify

Type B: Lamellae consist of degenerated cells. If the disturbance is more severe before the tooth erupts crack develops that is filled by surrounding cells.

Type C: Lamellae consisting of organic material. If crack appears after the tooth erupt it is filled by surrounding organic material, particularly originating from saliva.

Enamel tufts

These are small grass like structures (resembling tufts of grass) extending from the DEJ in to the enamel, occupying around 1/3rd or 1/5th of the total thickness of enamel. Tuft consist of hypocalcified enamel rods and interprismatic substance.

They extend in the direction of long axis of crown and hence they appear abundantly in horizontal sections and rarely in longitudinal section. Their appearance and their development is the consequence of spatial conditions in the enamel.

Enamel spindle

Occassionally odontoblastic process passes across the DEJ into the enamel and are termed enamel spindle. It originates from the odontoblastic process that extends into the enamel epithelium before hard substance are formed. Direction of enamel spindle corresponds to original direction of ameloblast i.e. at right angle to dentin.

Development of E. spindle

Before the enamel formation, some newly forming odontoblastic process push between adjoining ameloblasts and when enamel forms they remain trapped to form enamel spindle.

Enamel cuticle

Exactly this is not a part of enamel but a covering over a newly erupted tooth. This is typical basal lamina secreted by ameloblasts after the enamel formation is completed.

L.Q.A.3 Describe briefly about enamel organ

Ans. The embryonic oral cavity is lined by stratified squamous epithelium (oral ectoderm) At around 6th week of I.U life the oral ectoderm shows localised prolifretion resulting in horse shoe shaped band of tissue within mesenchyme called dental lamina. The ectoderm in certain areas of dental lamina continuous to proliferate and forms a knob like structure with mesenchyme called enamel organ. As the development further progresses the enamel organ goes through various morphological stages.

Following are the morphological stages:

- Bud stage
- Cap stage
- Bell stage
- Advance bell stage

Histologically following types of cells are distinguished:

- Outer enamel epithelium
- Inner enamel epithelium
- Stratum intermedium
- Stellate reticulum
- Dental sac follicle
- Dental papilla

Outer enamel epithelium

Outer enamel epithelium are couboidal cells that lines the convexity of enamel organ. Outer enamel epithelium have folds between them are present adjacent mesenchymal tissue carrying capillary loops which provide nutrition to enamel organ.

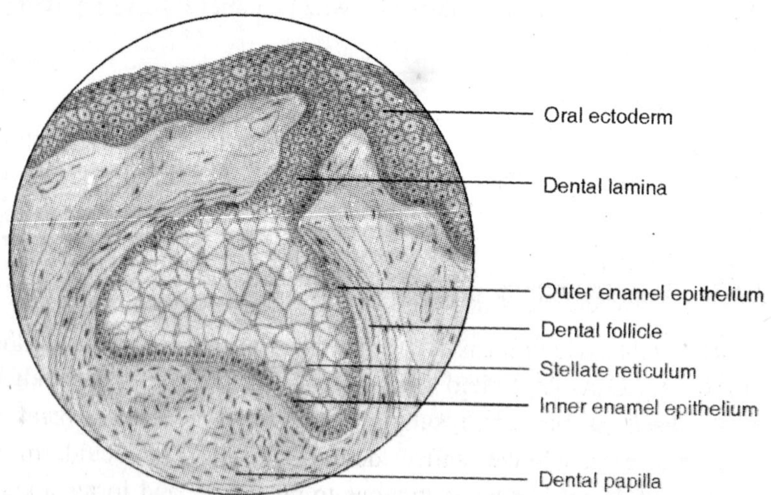

Fig. 3.7: Cap stage of tooth development (Ref. Fig. 3.2–Maji Jose)

Satellite reticulum

These are star shaped cells present between the outer enamel epithelium and inner enamel epithelium in cap stage but in bell stage it lies between outer enamel epithelium and stratum intermedium..

Stratum intermedium

Initially in the bud stage and cap stage these cells are not present in enamel organ. They appear in the bell stage. Stratum. intermedium are few layer of squamous cells that lies between inner enamel epithelium and stellate reticulum.

This layer of all cells shows great degree of metabolic activity and is essential for enamel formation.

Inner enamel epithelium

These are tall columnar cells that lines the concavity of the enamel organ. During the bell stage these cell proliferated and differential into ameloblasts. It also exert an influence on underlying connective tissue and initiates the formation of odontoblast.

Dental papilla

It is a part of condensed mesenchyme that is enclosed by invaginated enamel organ. In future dental papilla give rise to dental pulp and dentin.

Dental sac

Condensed mesenchymal tissue that surrounds the enamel organ is called dental sac or dental follicle. This tissue becomes denser and denser and more fibrous ultimately forms periodontal ligaments and also cementum.

Cervical loop

At the free border of enamel organ the outer and inner epithelial layers are continuous and reflected into one another as the cervical loop.

L.Q.A.4 Describe the life cycle of ameloblast

Ans. The life cycle of ameloblast is divided in to six stages.

1. Morphogenic stage
2. Organizing/Differentiating stage
3. Formative/Secretory stage
4. Maturative stage

5. Protective stage
6. Desmolytic

1. **Morphogenic stage:** Before the ameloblast completely differentiate and produce enamel under the influence of underlying mesenchyme they assume future DEJ and shape of crown.
   During this phase the cells are short and columnar with large oval nuclei centrally located. Golgi element are in proximal portion i.e. end adjacent to stratum intermedium. Mitochondnia and other cytoplasmic components are scattered through out the cells.
2. **Organizing/Differentiating stage:** During this stage the diffrentiating ameloblast becomes longer and elongated with the nucleus almost at proximal end. The golgi complex increases in volume and migrates to the central and distal end of the cell. Proximal part of cells shows large number of fine acidophilic granules. Thus the ameloblast become highly polarized with majority of organells situated at the distal end of cells.
   At the terminal phase of this stage dentin begins to appear. This cut down the original source of nutrition to ameloblast i.e. from papilla, and from then nutrition is supplied by the capillaries around or entering into the outer enamel epithelium.
3. **Formative stage/Secretary stage:** The ameloblast enter in the formative stage after the first layer of dentin has been formed. Thus for the begning of the enamel matrix formation it was necessary for epithelial cells to in close contact with the connective tissue of pulp during diffrentiation of the odontoblast and begeninig of dentin formation. Thus mutual interaction between two group of cells is very important in the organogenesis and histodifferentration.

Synthesis of enamel protein occurs in rough endoplasmic reticulum.

↓

Then it is passed to the golgi complex.

↓

In which it is condensed and packed into secretary granules.

↓

These granules migrate to distal end and their content in released against the newly formed mantle dentin.

As the 1st layer of enamel is formed the ameloblast migrate away from dental surface developing a short conical protection called "Tomes process".

4. **Maturative stage:** Once the full thickness of enamel matix is formed, it starts to mature. During the phase of enamel maturation the ameloblast slightly reduces in height and decrease in its volume and organelle content. During the maturation stage, qualitative and quantitative changes takes place in organic component of enamel and that the ameloblast may be involved in the selective removal of organic material.
5. **Protective stage:** As enamel maturation completed, the ameloblast ceases to be arranged in a well defined layer and can no longer be differentiated from the cells of the stratum intermedium. This cell layer covering the newly formed enamel in now called 'Reduced enamel epithelium'. It protects the newly formed mature enamel by separating it from connective tissue until tooth erupts.
6. **Desmolytic stage:** The reduced enamel epithelium proliferates and it seems to induce a atrophy of connective tissue so that the two epithelium, reduced enamel epithelium and oral epithelium come in contact and fuses. During this phase reduced enamel epithelium secreates certain enzyme that are able to destroy the connective tissue fibres.

L.Q.A.5 Describe in detail about amelogenesis

Ans. Enamel is a ectodermally derived hard/calcified tissue covering the anatomic crown of the tooth. The cells forming the enamel, ameloblast are derived from the inner enamel epithelium. Formation of enamel (amelogenesis) is divided into two processes

- Formation of enamel martix
- Mineralisation and maturating of enamel martix.

Although both the processes takes place simultaneously but for descriptive purpose are separated.

Formation of enamel matrix

As soon the 1st layer of dentin is laid down the inner enamel epithelium differentiate into ameloblast and start secreting enamel matrix. This matrix is partially mineralized so that the 1st formed enamel consist of approximatly 65% H_2O, 20% organic and 15% inorganic material. A thin layer enamel is formed around the predentin.This has been termed "Dentino enamel membrane".

Development of tomes process

These are the interdigitation of ameloblast into the enamel matrix and are named "Tomes process". At the time tomes process begin to form, terminal bars appears at distal ends of the ameloblast's separating the tomes process from the cell proper Structurally they are localized condensations of cytoplasmic substance closely associated with thickened cell membranes. In light microscope ameloblast covering the maturing enamel are shorter than the ameloblasts over incompletely formed enamel.

Mineralization and maturation of enamal

Mineralization of enamel matrix takes place in two stages.

1st stage: An immediate partial mineralisation occurs in the matrix segments and the interprismatic substance. Total mineral content at this stage is around 25% to 30% and is in the forms of crystalline apatite.

2nd *stage*: (Maturation) is characterized by gradual completion of materialization The process begins at the or cuspal or incisal height and progresses towards cervically, at the same time maturation begins at inner aspect first and progress towards the outer surface of enamel i.e. rod matures from depth to surface and sequence of maturing is from incisal/cuspal height to cervical region.

Maturation begins before the matrix has fully reached to its full thickeness. The advancing front of mineralization is first parallel to the DEJ and later to the outer enamel surface

Ultra structurally–maturation is characterized by growth of crystals. The ribbon shaped crystals increases in thickness more rapidly than in width. The organic matrix gradually becomes thinned providing space for growing crystals.

S.Q.A.1 Describe physical and chemical properties of enamel

Ans. Physical characteristics

Hardness: Because of high mineral content and crystalline arrangement enamel is the hardest calcified tissue in the human body. Provide the property to with stand the masticatory load, Enamel is brittle, therefore underlying resilient dentin is necessary.

Specific gravity: 2.8

Thickness: On the cuspal height = 2-2.5 mm thinning down to almost a knife edge at cervical line.

Permeability: it also act like a semipermeable membrane permitting complete or partial passage of certain molecules.

Colour: ranges from yellowish white to grayish white. Colour of enamel is determined by differences in the translucency of enamel.

Chemical properties:

Inorganic material: 96%

Organic substance: 4%

Inorganic material is similar to–apatite i.e. crystalline calcium phosphaste known as hydroxyappetite. Various other ions such as strontium, magnesium, lead and fluorides may be incorporated.

The chemical nature of organic substance has not been completely determined, but it is largely proteinaceous and contain some polysacharides.

S.Q.A.2 Enamel rods

Ans. It is a basic structural unit of enamel with highly organized pattern of crystal orientation. They are cylindrical in shape with an average diameter of around 4 μm. The diameter varies through out it length. Diameter increases from DEJ to the outersurface at a ration of 1 : 2

Enamel rods have somewhat tortuous courses towards surface. In longitudinal section the pattern of arrangement of rods is key hole or paddle shaped.

The number of enamel rod has been estimated ranging from 5 million in lower central incisors to 12 million in the upper 1st molar.

S.Q.A.3 Gnarled enamel

Ans. Over the cusps of tooth the rods appear twisted around each other in a complex manner known as gnarled enamel. This twisted arrangement creats an optical appearance. This also provides strength to the incisal and cuspal region.

S.Q.A.4 Incremental lines of Retzius

Ans. In ground section there appears a series of dark band illustrating the increasing pattern or successive apposition of enamel during its formation, In cross section they appears as concentric circles.

Its exact nature of its development is not known but it have been attributed to periodic bending of enamel rods, to variations in basic organic structure to physiologic calcification rhythm.

S.Q.A.5 Perkyimata

Ans. It is a external manifestation of the incremental lines of retzius appears as wave like grooves on external surface of enamel. They are continuous around a tooth and usually lie parallel to each other and to CEJ. There are around 30 perkyimata/mm at CEJ and gradually decreases to 10/mm near occlusal or incisal surface.

S.Q.A.6 Describe enamel cuticle

Ans. This a thin delicate membrane that covers the entire crown of the newly erupted tooth but is probably soon removed by mastication, It is also called "Nasmyths membrane"/primary enamel cuticle.

Under electron microscope, this membrane is a typical basal lamina found in most epithelium.

This basal lamina in apparently secreated by the ameloblasts after the enamel formation is completed.

S.Q.A.7 Dentino enamel Junction

Ans. It is a junction between the enamel and dentin established as two hard tissue begins to form. It has a scalloped profile with convexities towards the dentin. The dentinal surface is pitted in which rounded projections of enamel fits in it.

S.Q.A.8 Enamel tufts

Ans. It is a hypomineralised structure that arises from the DEJ and runs into enamel to about 1/3rd or 1/5th of total thickness of enamel. It resembles the tufts of grass and hence it is termed enamel tufts.

Their presence and development is consequence of spatial condition in the enamel during its formation.

S.Q.A.9 Enamel spindles

Ans. These are the extension of odontoblastic process that are rarely extended into the enamel across the DEJ. It is developed by the entrapment of odontoblastic process within the enamel.

Direction of enamel spindle corresponds to original direction of ameloblast i.e. right angle to dentin.

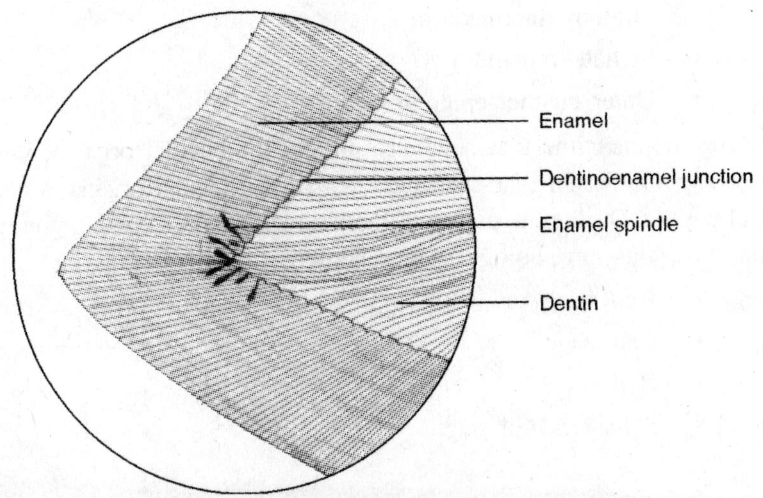

Fig. 3.9: Enamel spindle (Ref. Fig. 4.6–Maji Jose)

S.Q.A.10 Age changes of enamel

Ans.

(i) With age, the progressively worn away (i.e. attrition) in the occlusal surface and proximal contact points as a result of mastication

(ii) Teeth darken with age–it is either due to addition of organic material to enamel or due to deepening of dentin. Color seen through the thinning layer of enamel

(iii) Permeability decreases with age. Young enamel act as semi-permeable membrane but as age advances the pores diminishes as crystals acquire more ions and increase in size.

(iv) Composition of surface layer changes as ionic exchange occurs with the oral environments i.e. increase in fluoride content.

S.Q.A.11 Enamel organ

Ans. The ectoderm in certain areas of dental lamina continuous to proliferate and forms a knob like structure within the adjacent mesenchyme which is known as enamel organ. This is a primitive structure for the tooth development. Histologically following types of cells are distinguished

- Inner enamel epithelium
- Stratum intermedium
- Stellate reticulum
- Outer enamel epithelium

The mesenchyme that condense around the enamel organ is called dental sac/follide and that enclosed with in the enamel organs is called dental papilla. During the period of tooth development enamel organ goes through various morphologic stages namely.

- Bud stage
- Cap stage
- Bell stage
- Advance Bell stage

S.Q.A.12 Chemical composition of enamel

Ans. Enamel consist of organic and inorganic substance. Among which inorganic concentration is about 96 % and organic 4% Inorganic material is present in the form of hydroxy appetite i.e. crystalline calcium phosphate. Various other ions such as strontium, magnesium, lead and fluoride may be incorporated. The chemical nature of organic substance has not peen completely determined, but it is largely protienaceous and contain some polysaccharides.

S.Q.A.13 Hertwig's epithelial root sheath

Ans. Hertwigs root sheath is a continuation of cervical loop that consist of outer and inner enamel epithelium. It plays an important role in the formation of root. It influences (inner epithelium) the dental papilla to proliferate and differentiate in odontoblast in the radicular region. After a layer of dentin is laid down it fragments and may even persist in the future periodontal ligament as epithelial rest of mlassez.

S.Q.A.14 Ameloblast

Ans. It is eclodermally derived cell that give rise to enamel. The inner enamel epithelium proliferates and differentiate into ameloblast during the bell stage of tooth development under the influence of underling mesenchyme. The ameloblast passes through six stages

- Morphogenic stage
- Organizing stage
- Formative stage
- Maturative stage
- Protective stage
- Desmolytic stage

Initially the cells are short and coloumnar with oval nucleus located centrally later becomes elongated. The end of ameloblast towards stratum intermedium is called proximal end and end towards the dentin is called distal end.

In the late stage the nucleus is located towards the proximal end and all other cell organelles are towards the distal end

S.Q.A.14 Tomes process

Ans. The projections of the ameloblast into the enamel matrix have been termed Tomes process. Preciously it was believed that these processes were transformed into enamel, but recently it has been demonstrated that matrix synthesis and secretion by ameloblasts are very similar to the same processes occuring other protein secreting cells

It is developed when 1st structureless enamel layer is formed. The ameloblasts migrate away from the dentin surface and each ameloblast develops a short conical projection. The tomes process helps in creating rod-like structure in the enamel.

NOTES

4

Dentin

L.Q.A.1 Write briefly about types of dentin

Ans. Dentin is a ectomesenchymally derived hard calcified tissue that lies between the enamel and pulp in coronal region and between the cementum and pulp in reticular region.

Following are the different types of dentin

- Peritubular Dentin
- Intertubular Dentin
- Predentin
- Primary Dentin
- Secondary Dentin
- Tertiary Dentin
- Interglobular Dentin
- Sclerotic Dentin

Peritubular Dentin

It is a dentin that surrounds the dentinal tubules forming the wall for dentinal tubules. It is a part of primary dentin, highly mineralized i.e. 40% more than intertubular dentin. More accurate term for this dentin is "Intratubular dentin" because it forms within tubule there by narrowing the lumen.

Intertubular Dentin

The main body of dentin is composed of intertubular dentin. It is located in between the dentinal tubules.

About one half of its volume is organic material consist of tightly interwoven network of type I collagen fibrils.

Collagen fibres are roughly arrange of at right angle to the dentinal tubules and appatite crystals arranged parallel to the fibers. Ground substance consist of phosphoproteins proteoglycans, glycos-aminoglycans etc.

Predentin

Is a layer of dentin with variable thickness lies in the innermost portion (pulpal) of dentin. Thickness varies from 2-6 μm (orbans) 10-47μm (cates) It is a first formed dentin and is not mineralized, mainly consist of collagen and proteoglyeans. Its presence is important in maintaining the integrity of dentin since its absence may result in resorbtion of detain by odontoclasts.

Primary Dentin

It forms the bulk of the dentin. The outer layer of primary dentin is called "Mantle dentin" and inner layer of primary dentin is called circumpulpal dentin.

Mantle dentin: It is the 1st formed dentin lies jut adjacent to the DEJ of crown. It is about 20 μm thick.

Circumpulpal dentin: It forms the remaining bulk of dentin. Circumpupal is slightly more mineralized than mantle dentin.

Secondary Dentin

Dentin that formed after root completion. It is a narrow band of dentin bordering pulp. It is formed more slowly than primary dentin and contain fewer tubules. Secondary dentin does not form uniformly, appears in great amounts on the roof and floor of the coronal pulp chamber resulting in a symmetrical reduction in the size of pulp chamber. It is referred to as pulp recession.

Tertiary Dentin

It is also referred to as "Reactive, Reparative or Irregular dentin", produced in response to noxious stimuli. Unlike to primary and secondary dentin it is formed locally. The quality or architecture and quantity or degree of the tertiary dentin produced is related to the intensity and duration of the stimuli. Tertiary dentin is characterized by having fewer and more twisted tubules than normal.

Interlobular Dentin

It is a hypomineralisd zone between the globules that fails to coalesce. Normally mineralization of dentin begins in small globular areas called calcospherites which coalesce to from homogenous mass, But failure of calcosphaerite to fuse during dentin calcify action results in interlobular dentin.

Interlobular dentin is most frequently seen in circumpulpal dentin. There is only defect in mineralization the architecture remains uninterrupted.

Sclerotic Dentin

It is a protective response of dentin, that results in the obliteration of dentinal tubule by the deposition of minerals. The amount of sclerotic dentin increases with age.

L.Q.A.2 Describe in detail the microscopic structure of dentin.

Dentin is ectomesenchymally derived hard calcified structure that surrounds the pulp. It provides the bulk and general form of the tooth and is characterized by the presence of tubules throughout its length physically and chemically it resemble bone.

Microscopic structure

When the dentin is viewed microscopically several structural features can be identified.

These include the dentinal tubules, intra and inter tubular dentin. Areas of decalcified dentin are called interlobular dentin. Incremental growth lines, an area seen rarely in the root portion of the tooth known as granular layer of tomes and finally the cells of dentin odontoblast.

Dentinal tubules

These are small canal like structure that is filled with tissue fluid and odontoblastic process. It extends through the entire length of the dentin and follow 'S' shaped path. Dentinal fubules are tapered in outline measuring approx 2.5 μm diameter at pulp and 1.2 μm diameter at midway and it decreases further. These tubules also have lateral lobules which are termed as canaliculi.

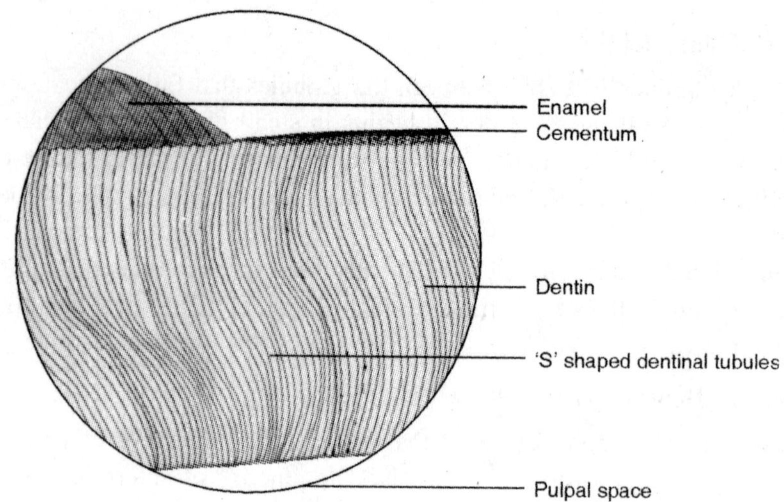

Fig. 4.1: 'S' shaped dentinal tubules (Ref. Fig. 5.1–Maji Jose)

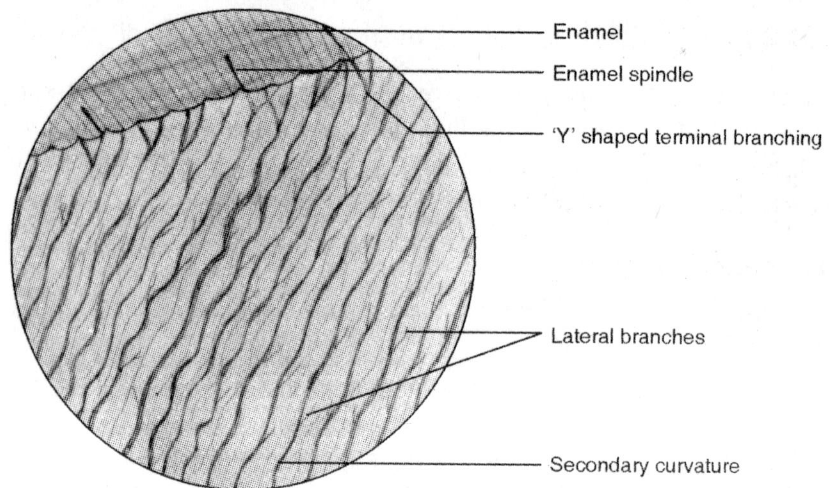

Fig. 4.2: Terminal branches & lateral branches of dentinal tubules (Ref. Fig. 5.2–Maji jose)

Peritubular dentin

It is part of primary dentin that surrounds the dentinal tubules and forms the wall. It is highly mineralized i.e. 40% more than intertubular dentin.

Intertubular dentin

It forms the main bulk of the dentin and is located in between the dentinal tubules. About one half of it volume is organic material is consist of tightly interwoven network of typs I collagen fibrils. Apatite crystal are arranged parallel to their long axis. Ground substance consist of phosphoproteins, proteoglycans, glycasaminoglycans, glyoproteins and some plasma proteins.

Interglobular dentin

It is a hypomineralized zone between the globules (mineralized area) fails to fuse enamel into a homogeneous mass. Interglobular dentin is most frequently seen in circumpulpal dentin. In these areas there in only defect in materialization but the architecture remains the normal.

Incremental lines: (von ebner lines) (contour lines of owen)

These are fine lines or striation run at right angle to the dentinal tubules reflecting the incremental or rhythmic pattern of dentin formation with alternating phase of activity and quiescence. These lines are best seen in longitudinal ground section of teeth. Distance between the line varies from 4-8 μm in the crown to much less in root.

Occasionally some of incremental lines are accentuated because of disturbance in the matrix and mineralized process Such lines are called "Contour lines of owen". In the decidous teeth and permanent 1st molar the dentin forms partly before birth, and partly after birth this prenatal and postnatal dentin is separated by an accentuated contour line known as neonatal line.

Tomes granular layer

A granular layer is seen in dry ground section under transmitted light is called tomes granular layer. These are empty space and appears dark when viewed in transmitted light.

Dead tracts

It is a area of dentin that appears dark when viewed in transmitted light. In this area the tubules are emptied either by complete retraction of odonoblast processes or death of odonoblast. The dentinal tubules than becomes sealed off. So that in ground section air filled tubules appears dark.

Sclerotic dentin

As a result of aging or from the mild irritation that cause obliteration of tubules due to the deposition of calcified material. It is harder, denser, less sensitive and more protective of the pulp against subsequent irritation.

Odontoblastic process: (Cells of dentin)

It is a cytoplasmic extension of odontoblast. It may or may not extend through the entire thickness of dentin. The processes are largest in diameter near the pulp and taper. Odontoblastic processes are composed of microtubules occasionally mitochondria, dense bodies resembling lysozome microvesicles and coated vesicles that may open to extracellular space.

Predentin

It is a layer of dentin with variable thickness lies in the innermost portion (pulpal) of dentin. Thickness varies from 2-6μm it is 1st formed dentin and is not mineralized mainly consist of collagen and proteoglycans.

S.Q.A.1 Dentinal tubules

Ans. Dentinal tubules are small canal likes spaces within the dentin filled with tissue fluid and is occupied by odontoblastic process. They extend through the entire thickness of dentin. They follow a 's' shaped path starting at right angle from pulpal surface the 1st convexity of this doubly curved course is directed towards the apex of the tooth. This 's' shaped curvature is less pronounced and least profound in root dentin. These curvatures are called primary curvatures. Other than these, there are minute, relatively regular secondary curvatures are also present. Dentinal tubules are tapered in outline measuring approximately 2.5 μm in diameters near pulp and 1.2 μm in midway and further decreases to DEJ

- There are around 20,000 tubule/mm^2 near enamel and 45000/mm^2 near pulp.
- These tubules also have lateral branches which are termed as canaliculi or microtubules. They may either reach to adjacent tubule or ends in the intertubular dentin.
- Sometime dentinal tubules may cross DEJ and enter into the enamel and is termed as "Enamel spindle".

S.Q.A.2 Types of dentin

Ans. Dentin is ectomesenchymally derived hard caleified tissue, that lies between the enamel and pulp in crown and between cementum, and pulp in root. Following are the different types of dentin.

Primary dentin: Forms the bulk of dentin and it consist of two type Mantle dentin lies adjacent to DEJ Circumpulpal dentin lies close to pulp

Secondary dentin: That forms after the root completion. Narrow band of dentin bordering pulp

Tertiary dentin: Reparative dentin produced in response to noxious stimuli

Peritubular dentin: It is a part of part of primary dentin that lines the dentinal tubule it is highly mineralized

Intertubular dentin: The main body of dentin is composed of intertubular dentin. It lies between the dentinal tubules

Predentin: It is a layer of dentin that is 1st formed and is not mineralized

S.Q.A.3 Predentin

Ans. It is a layer of dentin of varying thickness lies in the innermost portion of dentin. It is 1st formed and is not mineralized, mainly consist of collagen and peoteoglycons Its presence is important in maintaining the integrity of dentin. Since its absence may result in resorbtion of dentin by odontoblast.

S.Q.A.4 Circumpulpal dentin

Ans. It is a part of primary dentin that lies in the inner portion of primary dentin towards pulp.

S.Q.A.5 Secondary dentin

Ans. It is formed after the root completion. It is narrow band of dentin bordering the pulp. It is formed more slowly as compared to primary dentin and contain fewer tubules. Secondary dentin does not form uniformly, appears in great amounts on the roof and floor of the coronal pulp chamber resulting in asymmetrical reduction in the size of pulp chamber. It is referred to as pulp recession.

S.Q.A.6 Mantle dentin

Ans. The outer layer of the primary dentin is called mantle dentin. It is 1st formed dentin lies just adjacent to the DEJ of crown. It is about 20 μm thick.

S.Q.A.7 Neonatal line

Ans. An accentuated contoured line that separates the prenatal dentin and post natal dentin is called neonatal line.

In the deciduous teeth and permanent 1st molar the dentin partly forms before birth and partly after birth resulting in the development of neonatal line. This line reflects the abrupt change in the environment that occurs at birth.

S.Q.A.8 Tomes granular layer

Ans. A granular layer is seen in a dry ground section of root dentin adjacent to cementum. This is known a tomes granular layer. This zone is increases from the CEJ to the root apex and is believed to be caused by coalescing and looping of terminal portion of dentinal tubules.

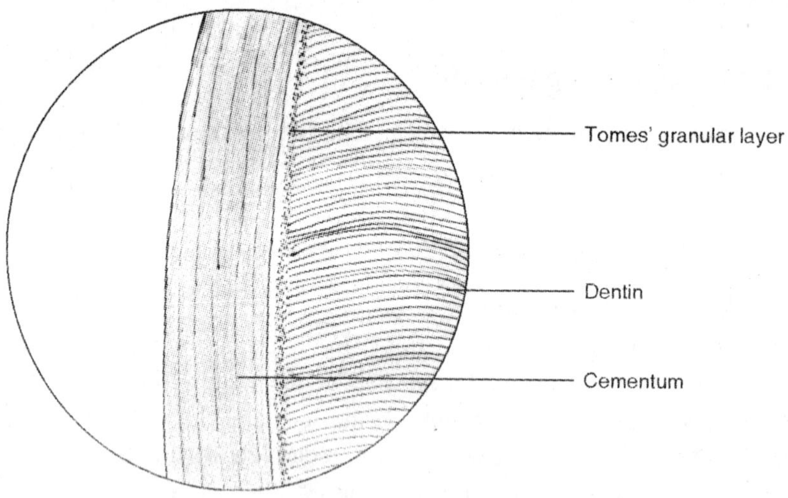

Fig. 4.3: Tomes' granular layer (Ref. Fig. 5.7–Maji jose)

S.Q.A.9 Dead tracts

Ans. Area of dentin associated with the death of the odontoblast.

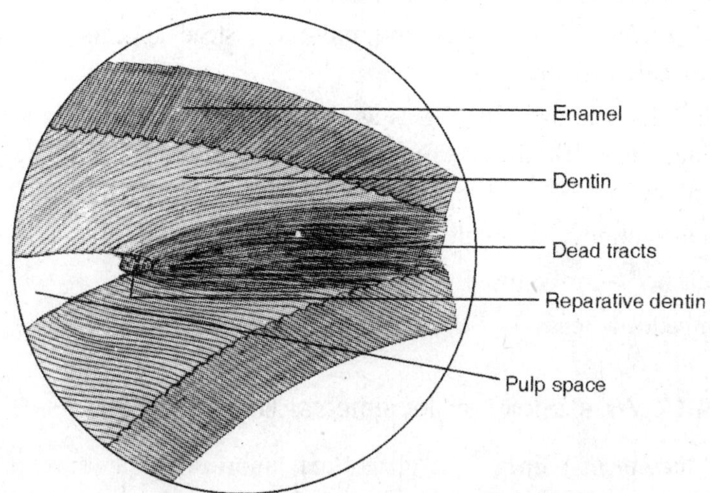

Fig. 4.4: Dead tracts (Ref. Fig. 5.8–Maji Jose)

These areas of dentin are called dead tracts. It extends from the external surface to the pulp. The tubules are empty and thus appears dark when ground section of dentin are viewed microscopically with transmited light. Dead tracts may results from moderate level stimuli or in the form of age related changes.

S.Q.A.10 Sclerotic dentin

Ans. Results from the aging or from the mild irritation that causes change in the composition of primary dentin. The peritubular dentin becomes wider, gradually filling the tubule with calcified material progressing pulpally from DEJ, These areas are harder, denser, less sensitive, and more protective of the pulp against subsequent irritations.

S.Q.A.11 Denticles/pulp stones

Ans. Are small discrete nodular calcified masses appearing either both the coronal and root portions of the pulp organ. They usually appears in otherwise normal teeth

Pulp stones may be either true or false type.

True denticles: Are similar to dentin in that they have tubules with odontobalastic process that formed them. True denticles are rare and are usually located close to apical foramen.

False denticles: They do not have tubules, instead appears concentric layers of calcified mass.

All pulp stone initially begins as small nodule but increases in size, sometimes may fill the entire pulp chamber. Further they are also classified as

Free—entirely surrounded by pulp

Attached—partly fused with dentin

Embedded—entirely surrounded by dentin.

S.Q.A.12 Write briefly on incremental lines in dentin

Ans. Incremental lines (von ebner line, imbrication) appears as fine lines or striations in dentin. They run at right angle to the dentinal tubules, reflecting incremental or rhythmic pattern of dentin formation with alternating phases of activity and quiescence. These lines are best seen in longitudinal ground section of dentin (Teeth)

Distance between the line varies from 4- 8 µm in the crown to much less in the root.

Occasionally some of incremental lines are accentuated because of disturbance in the martix formation and minerelization process such lines are called "Contour lines of Owen".

In the decidous teeth and permanent 1st molar the dentin forms partly before birth and partly after birth. This prenatal and postnatal dentin is separated by accentuated contour line which is known as neonatal line. This line reflects the abrupt change in environment that occurs at birth the dentin formed prior to birth is or better quality than formed after birth.

S.Q.A.13 Briefly explain dentin sensitivity

Ans. The dentin–pulp complex is sensitive and is difficult to explain why this complex is so sensitive. The overwhelming sensation appreciated by this complex is pain. Dentin is most sensitive at the DEJ and quite sensitive close to the pulp.

It is clear why the pulp is sensitive that is because pulp is well innervated for dentin sensitivity. Three mechanism or three theories are given.

(i) Direct neural stimulation theory
(ii) Transduction theory
(iii) Hydrodynamic theory (most popular)

Direct neural stimulation

According to this theory the stimuli directly reaches to the nerve ending in the inner dentin. It is thought that dentin is directly innervated by nerve.

Hydrodynamic Theory

The most popular and accepted theory. This theory proposes that noxious stimulus such as heat, cold, air blast result in the fluid movement through the dentinal tubules. This fluid movement either inward or outward results in distortion of local pulpal environment and is sensed by the local free nerve ending in the pluxes of Raschkow. Thus these never ending act as mechanoreceptors

Transudation theory

Odontoblasts are of neural crest origin and hence it is thought that it act as receptor as it may retain an ability of tansduce and propagate the impulse. But there is no neurotranmitter vesicles in the odontoblasts process to facilitate the synapse.

NOTES

5

Pulp

L.Q.A.1 Describe briefly about pulp

Ans. It is a mesenchymally derived loose connective tissue that lies inside the teeth or encircled by the hard structures of teeth. Anatomically pulp is divided in two parts.

Pulpchamber–pulp present in the crown portion of teeth,

Radicular pulp–pulp present in the root portion of teeth.

Histologically four distinct zones are described

- Odontoblastic zone
- Cell free zone (zone of weil)
- Cell rich zone (cell density is high)
- Pulp core

Cellular element of pulp

1. Odontoblast
2. Fibroblast
3. Undifferentiated mesenchymal cells
4. Defense cells

   (i) ***Fibroblasts:*** The most prominent cell of pulp is fibroblast. They are stellate or star shaped cells with extensive processes. Fibroblasts have abundant rough endoplasmic reticulum, mitchondria and other organelles that indicates the cells are active.

In young pulp–cells divide and active in protein synthesis. In older pulp cells appear rounded or spindle shaped with short process and exhibit fewer organelles termed fibrocytes.

(ii) ***Odontoblast:*** 2nd most prominent cells of pulp residing just adjacent to the predentin and the zone is called odontogenic zone of pulp. Cell body is columnar in appearance with large oval nucleus that fills basal part of cells. Adjacent to nucleus are rough-endoplasmic reticulum and golgi apparatus are present

Odontogenic process: It is an extension of the cell that enters into the dentinal tubules. Process does not contain endoplasmic reticulum but during early period it contain mitochondria and vesicles.

(iii) ***Undifferentiated mesenchymal cells:*** These are the primary cells in the very young pulp but few are seen in the pulp after root completion. They are polyhedral in shape with peripheral process and poses a large oval nucleous. They are believed to be totipotent cells and when needed they may give rise to odontoblast, fibroblasts, macrophages etc.

(iv) ***Defense cells:*** These are histocytes or macrophages mast cells and plasma cells. In addition to these there are blood vascular elements such as PMN, eosinophils, lymphocytes and monocytes

- Histocytes or macrophage are irregular shaped cell with short blunt processes. These cells are usually associated with small blood vessels and capillaries.
- The lymphocytes and eosinophils increases in number during inflammation.
- Plasma cells are seen during inflammation of pulp. Plasma cells function in the production of antibodies.

Inter cellular substance

The extracellular compartment of the pulp or matrix consist of collagen fibers and ground substance.

Ground substance: Ground substance of pulp resembles to that of any other loose connective tissue it is principally composed of glycosaminoglycan hyaluronic acid, chondritin sulfate, glycoprotein and water. It act as a support to the cells and act as a medium for the transport of nutrients from the vasculature to the cells.

Fibers

Fibers found in the pulp are principally type I and type II collagen in an approximately 55:45 ratio. As age advances the collagen content increases but ratio remains the same. The greatest concentration is seen in the most apical portion of the pulp

Vasculture and lymphatic supply

The pulp organ is extremely vascularized. Blood vessel enter and exist the dental pulp through the apical foramen. The arterioles occupy the central portion of the pulp and as they pass through the radicular portion of pulp give off smaller lateral branches. There is a extensive vascular network located below the odontoblastic layer in coronal portion. Some terminal capillary loops may extend upward between the odontoblasts to about the predentin. Efferent or drainage vessels of pulp are primarily composed of venules. Arteriovenous anastomoses have also been identified.

Lymphatic vessels also occur in pulp tissue. They arise as small blind thin walled vessels in the connal region.

Nerves

Abundant nerve supply in the pulp follows the distribution of the blood vessel. The majority of the nerves that enters the pulp are nonmyelinated. These nonmyelinated nerves are sympathetic in nature. These nerve bundles enter the apical foramen and pass along the radicular pulp to the coronal pulp where these fiber radiate peripherally to the parietal layer of nerves. This forms a network of nerves located adjacent to the cell rich zone and termed parietal layer of nerves or plexus of Rashkow. Nerve ending from parietal zone pass through the cell rich zone and cell free zones and either terminate, among or pass between the odontoblast to terminate adjacent to odontoblast processes at pulp predentin border on in dentinal tubules.

L.Q.A.2 Define pulp and describe the function of pulp

Ans. Pulp is mesenchymal derived soft (loose) connective tissue that is surrounded by a hard calcified structure of the tooth.

Functions of pulp:

1. **Inductive:** The primary role of pulp is to interact with oral epithelium and induces it to form dental lamina and enamel organ
2. **Formative:** The cells of pulp proliferate and differentrate into odontoblast which produces dentin that surrounds and protect the pulp
3. **Nutritive:** Pulp nourishes the dentin through the odontoblast and their processes and by means of the blood vascular system of pulp.
4. **Protective:** Pulp is innervated by nerves that respond with pain to the various stimuli. Nerves also initiate reflexes that control circulation time in the pulp.
5. **Defensive/Reparative:** Pulp has remarkable reparative property. It responds to irritation such as mechanical, chemical, thermal, bacterial etc. by producing reparative dentin and by mineralizing affected dentinal tubules.

   Invaded microorganisms are also removed by the pulp through inflammatory response and ultimately repair.

L.Q.A.3 Write briefly about age changes in pulp

Ans.

Cell changes

As age advances the cellular components decreases and fibre grows in number. The remaining cells are characterized by decrease in size and number of cytoplasmic organelles.

Fibrosis

In aging pulp there is increased accumulation of both diffuse fibrillar components and bundles of collagen fibres. Increase in fibres in the pulp organ is gradual and is generalized throughout the organ.

Vascular changes

Atherosclerotic plaque may appears in pulpal vessels. In other cases the outer diameter of vessel wall becomes greater as collagen fibres increases in the medial and advential layers.

Pulp stone

These are discrete, nodular calcified mass appearing in either or both coronal or radicular pulp. Pulp stones are classified as true or false

(a) ***True pulp stone:*** These are similar to dentin and have dentinal tubules

(b) ***False pulp stone:*** Does not exhibit dentinal tubules but appear instead, as concentric layers of calcified tissue.

They are also further classified as,

(a) *Free:* Totally surrounded by pulp

(b) *Attached:* Partly attached to dentin

(c) *Embedded:* Completely within the dentin

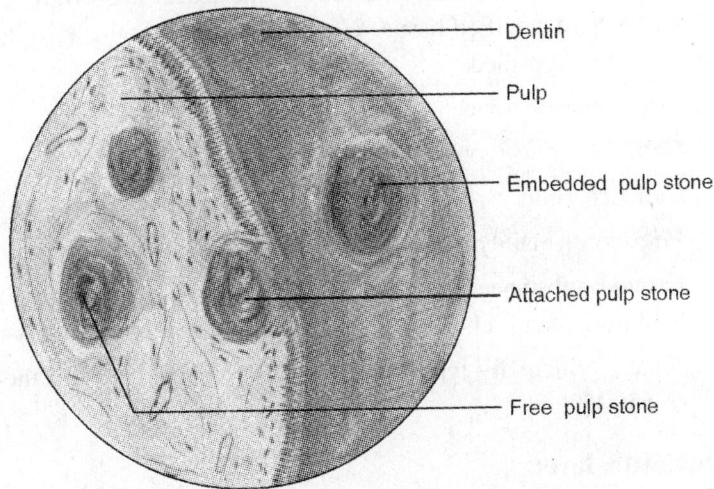

Fig. 5.1: Pulp Stones (Ref. Fig. 6.2–Maji Jose)

Diffuse calcification

Appears as irregular calcific deposits in the pulp tissue usually following collagenous fiber bundles or blood vessels Diffuse calcification usually affect the root canal where as denticles are seen more frequently in coronal pulp.

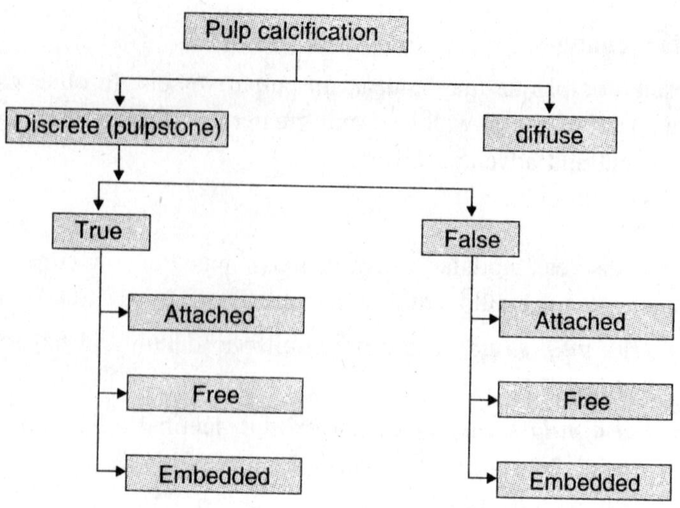

L.Q.A.4 Enumerate the structures present in the pulp and write in detail odontoblastic layer and its function

Ans. Pulp is soft connective tissue of mesenchymal origin and is surrounded by hard calcified tissue. When viewed histologically following structure are distinguished

- Odontoblastic zone
- Cell free zone (zone of weil)
- Cell rich zone
- Pulp core: mainly composed of blood vessels and nerves
- Ground substance. Principally composed of glycosominglycans hyaluronic acid, chondroitin sulphate, glycoproteins and water
- Fibres: principally type I and type III collagen fibres in the ratio of 55: 45

Odontoblastic layer

It is composed of odontoblast and lie just beneath the dentin Odontoblast are the second most prominent cell in the pulp & is present as a single layer lining the periphery of pulp and have process extending into the dentin. The cell has a body and process.

Body: The body of cells is columnar in shape with a large oval nuclei filling the basal part of the cells. Morphology of the odontoblast reflects the functional activity of the cell and ranges from an active synthetic phase to quiescence. Active cells are distinguished by possessing an open faced nucleus, basophilic cytoplasm and a negative Golgi zone.

Resting cell is flattened with relatively little cytoplasm and has more hematoxophilic nucleus.

Process: Odontoblastic begins at the neck of odontoblast where the cell gradually begins to narrow in diameter. A major change in cytology of odontoblast occurs at the junction between the cell body and it process. The process is devoid of major cell organelles but display abundant microtubules and filament arranged in a linear pattern. Occasionally mitochondria and vesicles may present.

Junctions

Many complex junction occurs between the adjacent odontoblasts. These junctions are gap junctions, zona occludens (tight junction) and zona adherens (desmosomes)

Life Span

Life span of odon oblast is believed to be equal to that of a viable tooth.

Function of odontoblast

Formative: Odontoblast forms dentinal matrix and function in its calcification to form dentin.

Nutritive: Pulp nourishes the dentin through odontoblast

Reperative: It respond to various noxious stimulus by producing reparative dentin and sclerotic dentin.

Conduction: Described by transduction theory. According this theory it is believed that odontoblasts have ability to transduce and propagate the impulse as it is originated from neural crest cells.

S.Q.A.1 Odontogenic region of pulp

Ans. It is a single layer of cells composed of odontoblast lies just beneath the predentin or occupics the periphery of the pulp. Odontoblast are the 2nd most prominent cells of pulp. Cell is composed of two part:

- Cell body
- Process

Cell body

Is columnar in shape with large oval nuclei. Active cells composed of large amount of basophilc cytoplasm and other organelles. Resting cell is flattened with relatively little cytoplasm.

Process

It is a cytoplasmic extension of odontoblast that extends into the dentin. Usually it is devoid of organelles but display abundant microtubules and filament arranged in a linear pattern. Occasionally mitochondria and vesicles may present.

S.Q.A.2 Age changes and clinical consideration of pulp

Ans.

Age changes

Cellular component decreases with increase in fiber component. Cells that remains are characterized by decrease in size and decrease in number of cytoplasmic organelles.

Fibrosis of the pulp with increased accumulation of diffuse fibrillar component and bundles of collagen fibres , It is gradual and is generalized.

Vascular changes

Atherosclerotic plaque may appear in vessels

Calcification of pulp: It may be diffuse or may be discrete in the form of denticles (pulpstone).

Clinical consideration

For all operative procedure the shape and extension of pulp is very important. In young persons pulp chamber is large and is hazardous to make deep cavity.

The shape, size and variation in pulp also necessary for the opening of pulp chamber during RCT or other pulpal procedures otherwise there may be great chance of perforation.

- Shape and location of apical foramen is an important aspect in the treatment of root canals. This prevents over instrumentation, perforation, and help in proper obturation.

- Accessory canal are rarely seen in radiographs and can not be treated endodontically but it does affect the success of endodontic therapy.
- Vitality of the pulp is depends upon the vascular supply but not on its nerve innervation

S.Q.A.3 Cellular elements of pulp

Ans. The cellular elements of pulp is primarily composed of

- Fibroblasts
- Odontoblasts
- Undifferentiated mesenchymal cell
- Defense cells
- Other inflammatory cells

Fibroblast

Are the prominent and numerous cell type of pulp & present in large no in the cell rich zone. Function of fibroblast is the formation of collagen fibres.

Odontoblasts

Is the second most important cell present in odontogenic layer. Cell has body and process that extends into the dentin.

Functions

Formative — Dentin formation

Nutritive — Through odontoblast pulp nourishes dentin

Reparative — Forms reparative dentin

Undifferentiated mesenchymal cells

These are totipoten tells Whenever require it proliferate and differentiate into odonoblast, fibroblast, or macrophages.

Defense cells

In addition to above cells there are defense cells in pulp and are histocytes or macrophage, mast cells and plasma cells.

Macrophage	—	phagocytosis
Mast cells	—	produces chemical mediators
Plasma cell	—	produces antibodies

Besides these inflammatory are also present neutrophils, ecsinophils basophils, lymphocytes and monocots. These cells emigrate from vessels in response to inflammation.

NOTES

6

Cementum

S.Q.A.1 Intermediate cementum

Ans. At cemento dentinal junction the both tissue are sometime is separated by tissue which does not exhibit features of either dentin or cementum and is called intermediate cementum.

It is believed that it develops by the entrapment of Hertwigs root sheath during rapid deposition of either dentin or cementum.

S.Q.A.2 Cementogenesis

Ans. Cementum formation is preceded by the dentin formation. Once the dentin is formed Hertwig's roots sheath fragment exposing the connective tissue to first form dentin. Cells from the connective tissue proliferate and differentiate into cementoblast which is responsible for cementum formation.

These cementoblast synthesize collagen and protein polysaccharides which forms the organic matrix of cementum. After some cementum matrix is laid down mineralization of cementum begins. Calcium and phosphate on present in tissue fluids are deposited into the matrix and are arranged in the form of hydroxyapatite

S.Q.A.3 Sharpey's fiber

Ans. It is a embedded part of principle fiber of periodontal ligament either in the cementum or in bone.

Sharpey's fiber in acellular cementum are generally mineralized completely whereas in cellular cementum they are partly mineralized at their periphery.

In bone sharpeys fiber occasionally passes uninterruptedly through the bone and continue as principle fiber of an adjacent PDL or they may mingle buccally and lingually with the fibres of periosteum covering the outer cortex

S.Q.A.4 Cellular cementum

Ans. It is a part of cementum that is incorporated with cellular element i.e. cementocyte. Cementocyte lie in the space called lacunae.

Cellular cementum is frequently formed on the surface of acellular cementum but it may comprise the entire thickness of apical cementum. It is because of this cellular cementum passive eruption of tooth is possible which helps in componsating the occlusal wear due to attrition.

S.Q.A.5 Cementoenamel junction

Ans. It is a relation between the cementum and enamel at the cervical region which variable

60% cases = Cementum overlaps enamel

30% cases = Cementum meets with enamel

10% cases = Cementum fails to meet

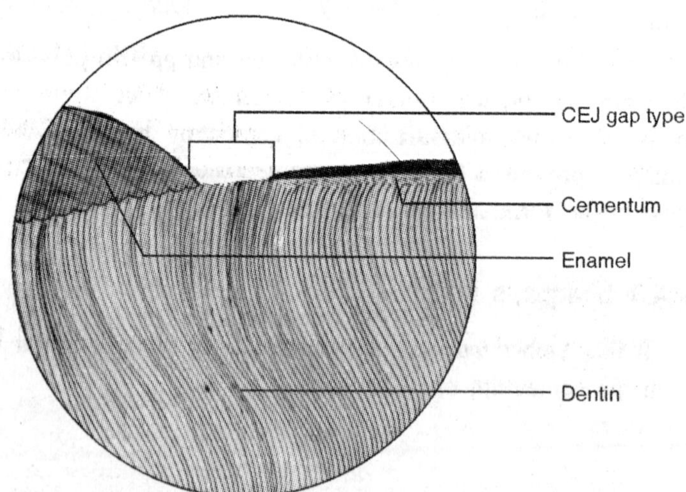

Fig. 6.1: Cementoenamel Junction- Gap type (Ref. Fig. 7.4–Maji jose)

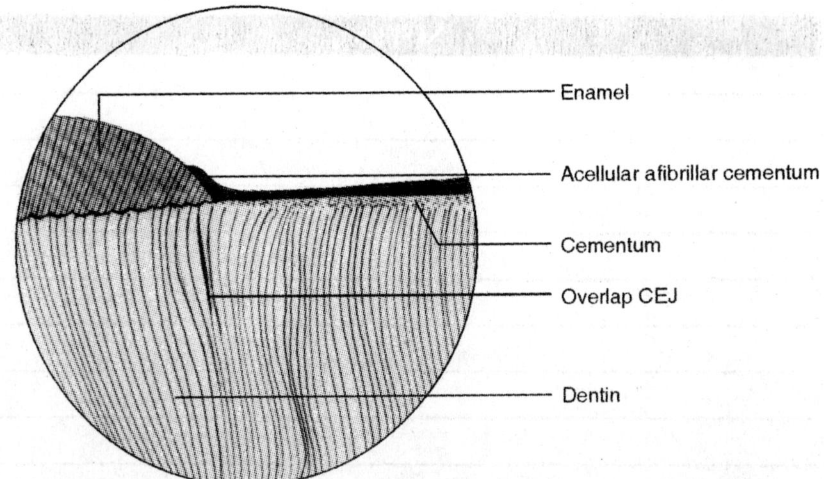

Fig. 6.2: Cementoenamel junction–overlap type (Ref. Fig. 7.5–Maji Jose)

Overlapping occurs when enamel epithelium degenerates at its cervical termination, permitting connective tissue to come in direct contact with enamel. Failure to meeting occurs when enamel epithelium in the cervical portion of root is delayed in its separation from dentin.

S.Q.A.6 Hypercementosis

Ans. Abnormal thickening of cementum is termed as hypercementosis. It may be diffuse affecting entire dentition or it may be confined to single tooth.

If hypercementosis improves functional qualities of cementum, is called cementum hypertrophy.

If hypercementosis is not related with increased function, is termed as cementum hyperplasia.

Localized hyper trophy: Spur or pronglike extension of cementum may be found. Usually found in teeth that are exposed to great stress

Localized hypercementosis: May observed in areas in which enamel drops have developed on the dentin.

Extensive hyperplasia of cementum is occasionally associated with chronic periapical inflammation. Thickening of cementum is often observed on teeth that are not in function.

NOTES

7

Periodontal Ligament

L.Q.A.1 Describe in detail the structure of periodontal ligament

Ans. The periodontal ligament is a connective tissue structure that surrounds the root and connects it with the bone, It serve as the attachment of the tooth to the alveolar bone. It primarily composed of bundles of continuous intermingling callagen fibres.

Structure of periodontal ligament

Structural component of periodontal ligament is broadly divided into following.

- **Extracellular substance**

  Fibres: collagen, oxytalan
- **Ground substance**

  Proleoglycans, glycoproteins
- **Cellular components**

Synthetic cells	: Fibroblast, Cementoblast, Osteoblasts
Resorptive cells	: Osteoclasts, Fibroclasts, Cementoclasts
Other cells present	: Epithelial rests of malasses, Mast cells, Macrophages, Undifferentiated cells

Extracellular substance fibres

The fibers of periodontal ligaments are made up of collagen and oxytalan

Collagen:

It forms the principal fibers of the periodontal ligament. Collagen present in periodental ligament is made up of predominantly of type I and type III collagen. Collagen fibers are arranged in bundles to form principal fibres. Principal fibers of the periodontal ligament are arranged in five particular groups, each group having a name as follows:

(i) **Alveolar crestal fibers:** The fiber bundles of this group radiate from the crest of the alveolar process and attach themselves to cervical part of the cementum.

(ii) **Horizontal group:** Located just apical to alveolar crestal fibers and runs perpendicular from the tooth to the alveolar bone.

(iii) **Oblique fiber:** Comprise the largest group run in coronal direction from the tooth to the bone

(iv) **Apical group:** Irregularly arranged and radiate from the apical region to the adjacent bone

(v) **Interradicular group:** Run from the crest of the interradicular septa to the furcation area of multirooted tooth.

The embedded part of principal fibers in the cementum and bone is called "Shorpey's fiber". The one section of principal fiber comes from bone and one from cementum and are joined in the mid region of the periodontal space giving a distinct appearance called "Intermediate plexus". This site provides site for rapid remodeling of fibers.

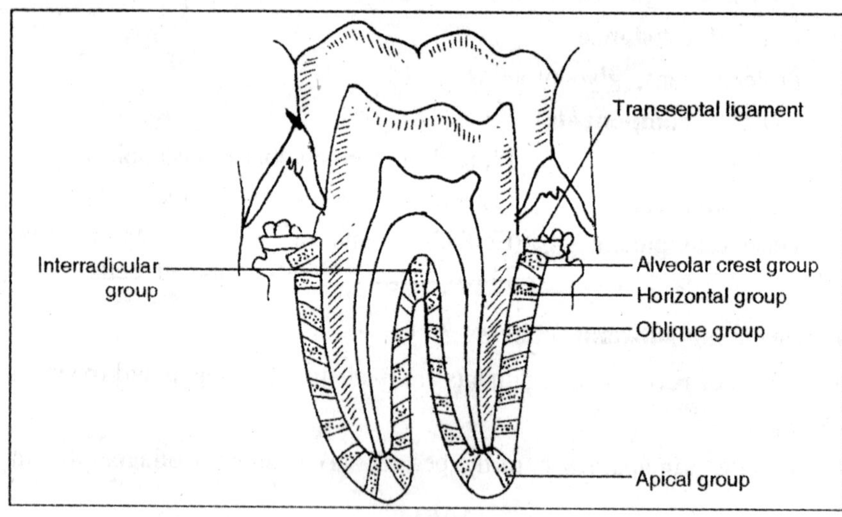

Fig. 7.1A

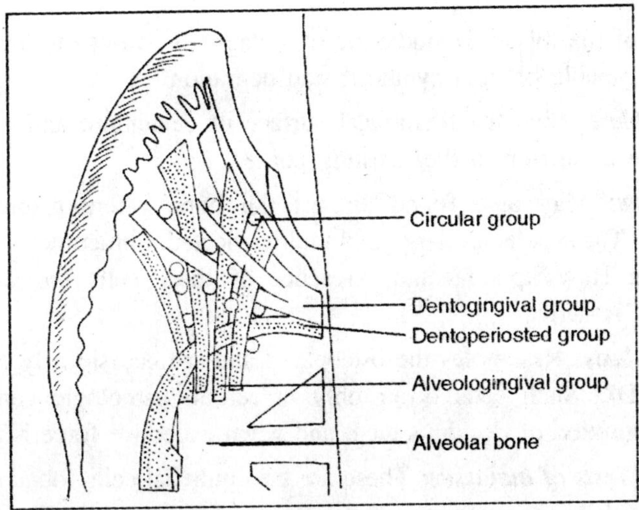

Fig. 7.1B

Oxytalan fibers

Although elastic fibers are found in the periodontal ligaments and are largely restricted to the wall of the blood vessels in humans. Oxytalan fibres are immature elastic fibre. Oxytalan fiber runs in axial direction one end in bone or cementum and other in blood vessel.

Ground substance

The space between fibers, cells, blood vessels and nerves is occupied by ground substance. It is made up of two major group of substances

- Proteoglycans
- Glycoproteins (fibronectin)

Cellular components

Osteoblast: The bone surface of ligament is lined by osteoblast. They are in various stages of differentiation depending upon functional state of the ligament.

Fibroblasts: Principal cell of periodontal ligament because of high rate of turnover in the PDL. Its constituents are constantly being synthesized, removed and replaced. This turnover is achieved almost exclusively by the fibroblast.

Function of fibroblast: Remodelling of collagen is achived by fibroblast, which is capable of both synthesis and degration.

Cementoblast: Line the ligamental surface of cementum and are most often seen in section in their resting phase.

Osteoclasts: May also found against the bone where resorption is occurring. These cells are large and multinucleated. Sometimes they may present in Howship's lacunal. Presence of these cells indicates that resorption is active.

Cementoclasts: Resembles the osteoclasts and are occasionally found in normal PDL. Such cells occur only in certain pathologic conditions, during resorption of decidous teeth and when excessive force is applied.

Epithelial rests of malassez: These are the epithelial cells found close to cementum. It is the remnants of the Hertwigs root sheath. They persist as a network, strands islands or tubule like structures near and parallel to root surface.

Undifferentiated mesenchymal cells: These are the important cellular constituents of the PDL. They are located in perivascular location. They are single progenitor cells. When require they proliferate and differentiate into fibroblast, osteoblast and cementoblast.

Structures present in connective tissue

- Blood vessels
- Lymphatic
- Nerves
- Cementicles

Blood vessels

Blood vessels of PDL are derived from 3 sources

- From apical vessels
- From intraalveolar vessels
- From gingival vessels

Lymphatics

Lymphatic vessels follow the path of blood vessels, provides lymphatic drainage of PDL

Nerves

Are usually associated with blood vessels and enters into the PDL. These nerve fibers are either myelinated or non-myelinated. Large fibers end in variety e.g.. knob like, spindle like and meissner like.

Cementicle

These are small irregular shaped calcified structures present in PDL. Usually found in older individuals and they may remain free in connective tissue or they may attached to cementum.

S.Q.A.1 Describe functions of PDL

Ans.

Function of PDL are as follows

1. Mechanical
2. Formative
3. Nutritive
4. Sensory

1. **Mechanical function:** Are to attach the tooth to the bone and provide a cushion that will absorb those force directed on teeth during mastication or other para functional force. In addition principal fibers transmit tension force to the alveolar bone.
2. **Formative function:** Is carried out by the cells present in the PDL

   Cementoblast: Throughout life of the tooth cementoblast are continuously forms cementum

   Fibroblast: Remodeling of collagen

   Osteoblast: Bone formation
3. **Nutritive:** It is provided by the blood vessels present in the PDL. These blood vessels supply anabolites and other substance required by the cells of ligaments
4. **Sensory function:** The nerves present in the PDL provide sensory function. Both pain and proprioceptive mechanism is possible. Through proprioceptive mechanism, it allows to detect the application of most delicate forces on the teeth.

S.Q.A.2 Describe briefly about principle fiber of PDL

Ans. The periodontal ligament is the connective tissue that surrounds the root and provide attachment of the tooth to the alveolar bone. It consist primarily of bundles of continuous intermingling collagen fibers arranged in bundles are referred to as "Principal fibers". The principal fibers are predominantly formed by the Type I and type III collagen.

Principal fibers are arranged in five particular groups

(i) ***Alveolar crest group:*** These runs from the crest of alveolar process to cervical part of cementum.

(ii) ***Horizontal group:*** Located just apical to alveolar crestal fibers and runs perpendicular from the tooth to the alveolar bone.

(iii) ***Oblique fiber:*** Comprise the largest group runs in coronal direction from the tooth to the bone.

(iv) ***Apical group:*** These are irregularly arranged and radiate from the apical region to the adjacent bone. It is absent in the young tooth where the apex is yet to complete

(v) ***Interradicular group:*** Fibers run from crest of interradicular septa to the furcation area of multi rooted tooth.

The part that is embedded in the bone or in cementum is termed as sherpey's fiber. One section of principal fibers comes from the cementum and other section from bone and are joined in the mid region of the periodontal space giving a distinct aperance and is called Intermediated plexus. This site provides site for rapid remodeling of fiber

S.Q.A.3 Rest of malassez

Ans. These are epithelial cells found close to the cementum. It is the remanants of Hertwig's root sheath. They persist as a network, strands, islands or tubular like structure near and parallel to root surface. These cells have no known function, but their presene can lead to the formation of dental cyst when PDL get infected.

S.Q.A.4 Cells of PDL

Ans. The two basic components of PDL are Cellular and Fibers:

Cellular components

(i) **Synthetic cells**

- Osteoblast
- Fibroblast
- Cementoblast

(ii) **Resorptive cells**

- Cementoclast
- Osteoclast
- Fibroclast

(iii) **Other cells**

- Epithelial cell
- Undifferentiated mesenchymal cells
- Macrophages
- Mast cells

Fibroblast are principal cells of PDL and their function is remodeling of collagen.

Bone cells are osteoblast and octeoclast, they lie against the bone.

Osteoclast – bone formation

Osteoclast – bone resportion. Presence of osteoclast indicate active resorption

Cementoblast and cementoclast lie against cementum. Cementoblast often seen in resting phase. Cementoclast are resorptive cells and are occasionally present. These cells (cementoblast) occurs only in abnormal conditions.

Epithelial cells (malassez) are remnants of hertwig's root sheath. Undifferentiated mesenchymal cells: These are totipotent cells (progeniter cells). They differentiate into fibroblast, osteoblast cementoblast etc.

S.Q.A.5 PDL

Ans It is a soft fibrous connective tissue that surrounds the tooth and serve as the attachment of the teeth to the bone

Structural component

1. ***Extacellular***

   Fiber – Collagen, Oxytalion

   Proteoglyeans, glycoproteins

2. ***Cellular components***

Synthetic	Resorptive
• osteoblast	• fibroblast
• fibroblast	• osteoclast
• cementoblast	• cementoclast

Other cells are: epithelial rest of malassez, progeniter cells, mast cells and Macrophage.

Fibres

Principal fibers of PDL are primarily made of type I and Type III collagen and arranged in bundles.

Principal fibers are grouped in five groups

- Alveolar crest group
- Horizontal group
- Oblique group
- Apical group
- Interradiculor group

Function of PDL:

1. ***Formative:*** it is carried out by cells of PDL

   Cementoblast: cementum formation

   Fibroblast: collagen remodeling

   Osteoblast: bone formation

2. ***Nutritive:*** Blood vessels present in the PDL provides nutrition to the cells present in PDL

3. ***Mechanical:***

   Provide attachment of teeth to bone

   Absorb force directed on teeth

   Transmit force to the bone from teeth

4. ***Sensory:*** Nerves present in PDL provide sensory function. Both pain perception and proprioceptive mechanism it possible.

S.Q.A.6 Periodontium

Ans. The tissue that surrounds and support the teeth is known as the periodontium. It composed of following structure

Two clacified structure

1. Cementum
2. Alveolar bone

Two soft tissue

1. Gingiva
2. Periodontal ligament

The periodontium is attached to the tooth by cementum and the bone of jaws by alveolar process/bone.

S.Q.A.7 Oxytalan fibres

Ans. These are immature elastic fibers They run in oblique direction between the walls of blood vessels in the ligament and cementum or at right angle to principle fibres

Function

Provide anchorage for blood vessels during distortion of the ligament in function.

NOTES

8

Maxilla and Mandible

L.Q.A.1 Write briefly about Meckels cartilage

Ans. It is a cartilage of 1st arch. It plays an important role in the formation of mandible but it does not have direct contribution in formation, it only provides framework for developing mandible.

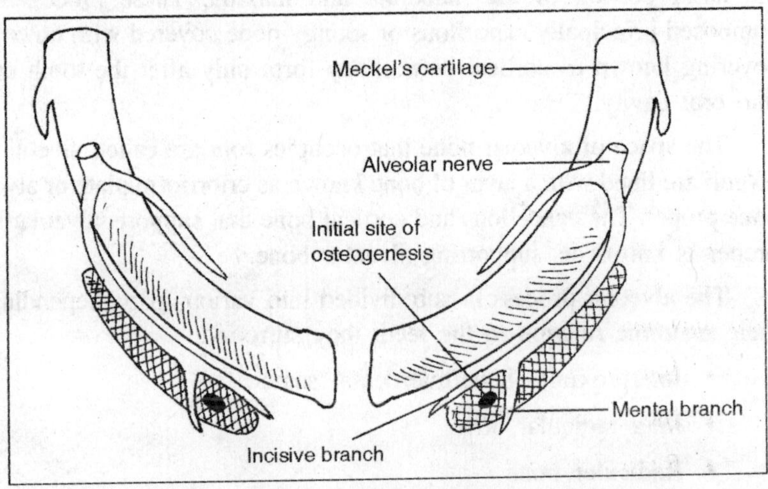

Fig- 8.1 Site of intial osteogenesis related to mandible formation

At the 6th week of development this cartilage extends as a solid hyaline cartilaginous rod, surrounded by a fibrous capsule, from the developing ear (otic capsule) to the midline (symphysis region). They are two in number on either side, but they remain separate in the midline by a thin band of mesenchyme. It is closely related with mandibular nerve.

Mesenchymal condensation, ossification and spread of new bone formation all occurs on the lateral aspect of cartilage. After the rudimentary mandible is formed (10 week around) the cartilage resorbed leaving behind some remanent that develops into

- Sphenomandibular ligament
- Incus, malleus
- Mental ossicles
- Spine of sphenoid
- Sphenomandibular ligament
- Sphenomelleolar ligament

S.Q.A.1 Alveolar bone

Ans. The alveolar bone is made up of bony processes that project from the basal portion of the mandible and maxilla. These processes are composed principally cancellous or spongy bone covered with outer hard covering known as cortical bone. They form only after the tooth erupts into oral cavity.

The space of alveolar bone that occupies root are called alveoli. The alveoli are lined with a layer of bone known as cribriform plate or alveolar bone proper. The cancellous and cortical bone that supports alveolar bone proper is known as supporting alveolar bone.

The alveolar process in sub divided into various parts depending on their anatomic relation to the teeth they surround.

- Interproximal bone/Interdental septa
- Inter radicular bone
- Radicular bone

S.Q.A.2 Bundle bone

Ans. Bundle bone is that part of alveolar process in which the fibres of the PDL are inserted and continue as a sharpays fiber. It is characterized by scarcity of the fibrils in the intercellular substance. These fibrils are arranged at right angle to saerpeys fiber. Bundle bone consist more calcium salts per unit area than any other type of bone. Such area appear dense radioopaque in radiograph and termed lamina dura.

S.Q.A.3 Howship Lacunae

Ans. Resorption of bone is primarily related to the cell known as osteoclast found in the concavities of bone surface called Howship lacunae. Howship lacunae are shallow, hollowed out depression occupied by osteoclast, which is created by themselves.

S.Q.A.4 Reversal line

Ans. Reversal line mark the change from bone resorption to bone deposition. After a period bone resorption ceases and a new bone is apposed on the old. The scalloped outline of Howships lacunae that turn their convexity toward the old bone, remains visible, which in termed as Reversal line.

NOTES

NOTES

9

Oral Mucous Membrane

L.Q.A.1 Describe briefly keratinized oral mucosa

Ans. It is the moist lining of the oral cavity that extends anatomically between skin (i.e. vermellian border of lip) and intestinal mucosa. It consist of two parts

1. Covering epithelium
2. Underlying connective tissue

   Oral mucosa may be divided into three major types

   - Masticatory mucosa
   - Lining mucosa
   - Specialized mucosa

   It can also be divided as:

1. *Keratinized:*

   Masticaltory mucosa. Vermilion border of lip

2. *Non keratinized:*

   Lining mucosa Specialized mucosa

Keratinized mucosa

It is that part of oral mucosa that is present on the gingiva and hard palate. Basically the oral mucosa membrane is made of two components.

- Outer epithelium
- Underlying connective tissue

In keratinized mucosa the overlying epithelium is keratinized. Keratinized oral epithelium has four cell layers.

- Basal cell layer/stratum basalae
- Spinous layer/stratum spinosum
- Granular layer/stratum granulosum
- Cornified layer/stratum corneum

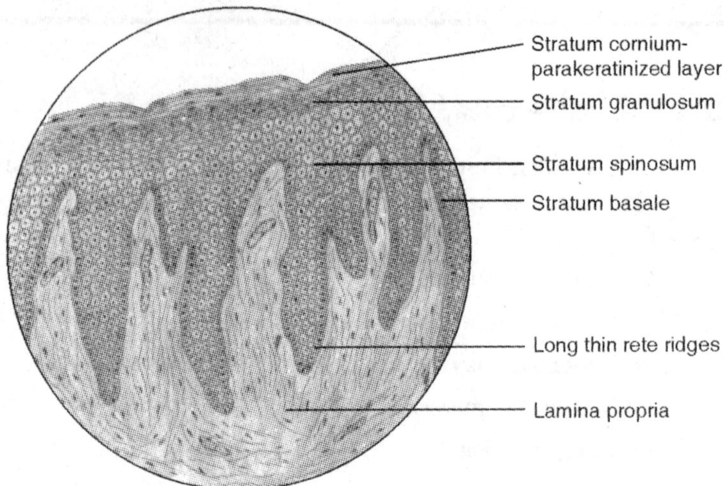

Fig. 9.1: Gingiva (Ref. Fig. 10.2–Maji Jose)

Oral epithelium

Stratum basalae

Single layer of cells containing cuboidal or columnar cells. These cells contain bundles of tonofibrils. The basal cells about on basal lamino by a special structure called hemidesmosomes and with each other by desmosomes

Stratum spinosum (Prickle cell layer)

These are large ovoid cells containing conspicuous tonofibril bundles. Adjacent cells are joined with each other through desmosomes.

Stratum granulosum

The most characteristic feature of keratinized epithelium is the appearance of keratohyaline granules in the granular cell layer. Keratohyline granules intimately associated with the tonofibrils. The protein that makes the bulk of granule is called flaggrin. As the cells of this layer reach superficially sudden change in their appearances occurs. It losses it organelles including the nuclei and granules disappears.

Stratum corneum

A superficial layer of keratinized mucosa which is dehydrated and extremely flattened layer is acidophilic. Ultrastructurally this layer is composed of densely packed filaments developed from tonofilaments.

The cells of the epithelium that ultimately keratinizes are called keratinocytes.

Connective tissue

Lamina propria

The connective tissue component of oral mucosa is called lamina propria. It is divided into two layers the superficial papillary layer and deeper reticular layer. In the papillary layer there is epithelial ridges and in this the collagen fibers are thin and loosely arranged. In reticular layer the collagen fibers are arranged in net like fashion. Lamina propria consist of cells, blood vessels neural elements and fibres embedded in an amorphous ground substance.

L.Q.A.2 Classify oral mucosa and describe in detail about masticatory mucosa

Ans.

Classification on Functional Criteria

(i) Masticatory mucosa: Gingiva, Hard palate

(ii) Lining or reflecting mucosa: lip, cheek, vestibular fornix, alveolar mucosa, floor of mouth and soft palate

(iii) Specialized mucosa dorsum of tongue and taste buds

Further it is also divided into following

(i) Keratinized areas

- Masticatory mucosa
- Vermilion border of lip

(ii) Non keratinized area.
- Lining mucosa
- Specialized mucosa

Masticatory mucosa

It is a keratinized and it covers those area of oral cavity such as the hard palate and gingiva, that are exposed to compressive and shear forces. Masticatory mucosa is immovably attached to the underlying structure. The overlying epithelium is similar in both hard palate and gingiva it may be orthokerotinized or parakeratinized. But there is little variation in lamina propria and submucosa.

Hard palate

Covering epithelium: Thick orthokeratinized (also parakeratinized) stratified squamous epithelium. Epithelium of hard palate have transverse palatine ridges (rugae)

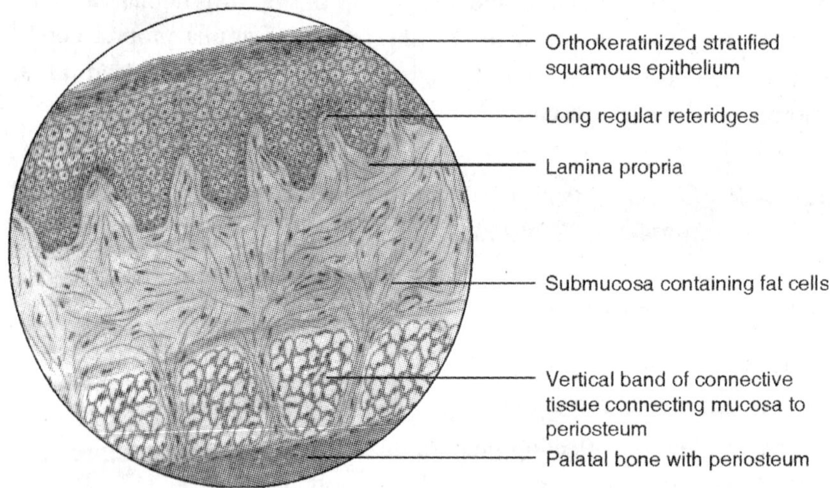

Fig. 9.2: Anterolateral area of palate (Fatty zone) (Ref. Fig. 10.3–Maji Jose)

Lamina propria: Shows long papillae and numerous thick dense collagenous connective tissue, which is not highly vascularized. Lamina propria and periosteum is present below the epithelium below the palatine raphe.

Submucosa: It is extend between the palatine gingiva and mid palatine raphe Despite this wide extension of submucosa the mucous membrane is immovably attached to the periosteum. Submucosa is dense collagenous In the anterior region submucosa contain adipose tissue, where as the posterior part it contain salivary glands.

Because of varying structures of submucosa, various region of hard palate differ from each other. Following zones can be distinguished

- Gingiva region adjacent to teeth
- Palatine raphe, also known as the median area extending from incessive papilla
- Anterolateral area or fathy zone
- Posterolateral area or glandular zone

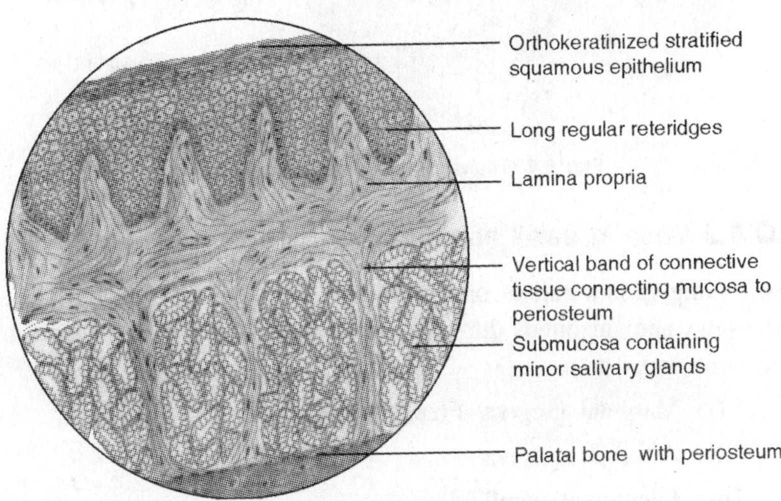

Fig. 9.3: Posterolateral region of palate (Glandular zone) (Ref. Fig. 10.4–Maji Jose)

Gingiva

It is part of mucosa that immediately surrounds the erupted tooth. Gingiva extends from the dentogingival Junction to the alveolar mucosa

Epithelium: It is thick, orthokeratinized or parakeratinized stratified squamous epithelium. Overlying epithelium often shows stippling. This is due to high retepegs of the lamina propria.

Lamina propria: It is dense collagenous with long narrow papillae. There is no submucosa, mucosa in firmly attached to the cementum and periosteum of alveolar bone by collagen fibers.

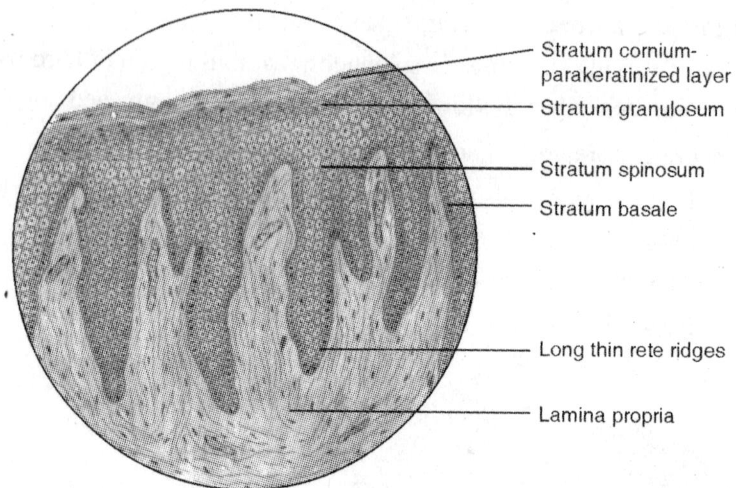

Fig: 9.4 Gingiva (Ref. Fig. 10.2–Maji Jose)

L.Q.A.3 Write in detail about gingiva

Ans. Gingiva is a part of oral mucosa that covers the alveolar process of the jaws and surrounds the neck of the teeth. Gingiva is divided into three contiguous areas

(i) Marginal gingiva/ Free gingiva

(ii) Attached gingiva

(iii) Interdental papilla

(i) **Marginal gingiva:** Most coronally positioned portion of gingiva. It is not attached to the bone. The dividing line between free gingiva and attached gingiva is called free gingival groove. A shallow 'V' shaped notch appears between the free gingiva and tooth, which is known as gingival sulcus.

(ii) **Attached gingiva:** Just apical to the free gingiva, part of the gingiva that is firmly bound to the underlying bone is called attached gingiva Below it is demarcated from the oral mucosa by mucogingival junction.

(iii) **Inter dental papilla:** Portion of gingiva located in the interproximal space created by adjacent teeth. In mesiodistal direction the shape of papilla is triangular. In three dimensional view it appears as tent shaped.

The oral and vestibular corner of the papilla are high and central part is like a valley. This central concave area is called Col and is lined by nonkeratinzed epithelium.

Surface characteristic or clinical appearance

Normally the color of gingiva is corol pink but it depends upon the following

- Degree of keratinization
- Thickness of epithelium
- Vascularity

Surface of gingiva is stippled

HISTOLOGY

Epithelium

It is stratified squamous epithelium. The epithelium that covers the oral or outer surface of gingiva is either keratinized or parakertinized. The epithelium that lines the gingival sulcus is thin non keratinized and without retepegs.

Junctional epithelium is part of gingival epithelium that forms a collar like band around teeth, and is non keratinized.

- The epithelium of gingiva shows four layers of cells.
- *Stratum basalae* - Deepest cuboidal cells
- *Stratum spinosum* - Polygonal cells
- *Stratum granulosum* - Flattened cells with prominent keratohyaline granules
- *Stratum corneum* - Superficial layer.

Connective tissue (lamina propria)

The connective tissue layer of gingiva is composed of

(i) Collagen fibers

(ii) Ground substance

(iii) Cells

(iv) Blood vessels

(v) Nerves.

Collagen fibers of gingiva are arranged following major groups.

(a) **Dentogingival:** From cervical cementum into lamina propria of gingiva

(b) **Alveologingival:** From alveolar crest to the lamina propria of gingiva

(c) **Circular:** Circle the tooth and interlacc with other fiber

(d) **Dentoperiosteal:** from cementum into the periosteum of the alveolar crest

Cells: following are the prominent cells found in the connective tissue of gingiva plasma cells, fibroblast, mast cells, lymphocytes.

L.Q.A.4 Describe about lining mucosa

Ans. It is that part of oral mucosa that covers the lip, cheek, vestibular fornix, floor of mouth, alveolar process and soft palate, The lining mucosa in characterized by thick nonkeratinized epithelium and a thin lamina propria. There is a variation in the submucosa of various zones of lining mucosa.

Epithelium: Thicker, non keratinized. The surface is thus flexible and able to withstand stretching.

Lamina propria: Is thicker and contains fewer collagen fibers that follow a more irregular course, also consist of elastic fibers. The lining mucosa where it covers the muscle, it is attached by a mixture of collagen and elastic fibre

Lip and cheek: Epithelium is stratified squamous, keratinized

- Lamina propria consist of dense connective tissue and has short, irregular papillae
- Submucosa attached the mucosa firmly to underlying muscle by collagen and elastin submucosa contains fats minor salivary gland and some times submucosa glands.

Alveolar mucosa

Epithelium: Thin non keratinized stratified squamous epithelium

Lamina propria: have short papillae and consist of elastic fibers. Submucosa in loses connective tissue, containing thick elastic fibers attaching to periosteum of alveolar process. It may contain minor salivary gland.

Inferior surface of Tongue (ventral surface)

The epithelium in relatively thin, non keratinized stratified squamous epithelium Lamina propria is thin with numerous short papillae and some elastic fibres. Few minor salivary glands may also present. Submucosa is thin and irregular and binds the mucous membrane tightly to tongue musculature.

Floor of Mouth

The oral mucosa in the floor of mouth is relatively very thin and is loosely attached to underlying structure to allow the free movements of tongue. Lamina propria is are short. The submucosa contain adipose tissue and minor salivary glands.

Soft Palate

The mucosa membrane of soft palate is highly vascularized and reddish in color. Epithelium is thin nonkeratinized lamina propria is thick with numerous short papillae. Distinct layer of elastic fibers submucosa is relatively loose and contains minor salivary glands It also contain taste buds.

L.Q.A.5 Describe microscopic and macroscopic structure's on dorsal surface of anterior 2/3rd of tongue

Ans. Tongue is a muscular organ which function as on organ of taste, degulitation and speech and also assist in mastication. The superior or dorsal surface of tongue is rough and irregular due to the presence of various taste bud. A 'V' shaped line divides the tongue into antenior 2/3rd or body and posterior 1/3rd or base of tongue. Anterior 2/3rd of tongue have various fine, pointed, cone shaped papilla gives a valvet like appearance to the tongue's dorsal surface

Histology

Mucous membrane of the tongue in specialized mucosa.

Covering epithelium

It is thick, keratinized and nonkeratinized, stratified squamous epithelium forming various types of papilla, some of the papilla bears taste buds

(i) **Circumvallate papillae:** It is present just anterior to the sulcus teminalis and are 8 to 12 in number. They are large and circular and bounded by a circular furrow.

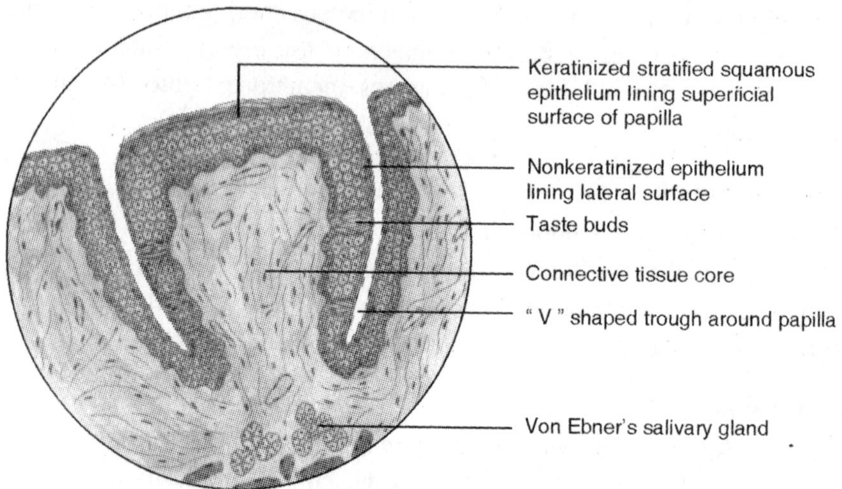

Fig. 9.5: Circumvallate papilla (Ref. Fig.10.7–Maji Jose)

Microscopically: Each papillae has a central core of connective tissue surrounded by a keratinized epithelium on the lateral surface they contain numerous taste buds. Associated with each papillae are some serous gland (von ebner) their duct opens in the trench–like furrow around papilla

(ii) **Filliform papillae:** cover the entire anterior part of the tongue and consist of bone shaped structure

Microscopically: it consist of core of connective tissue covered by a keratinized epithelium

(iii) **Fungi form papillae:** Anterior portion of the tongue contain both filliform and fungiform papillae. Single fungi form papillae are scattered between the numerous filiform papillae at the tip

Microscopically: They are smooth, round structures with central connective tissue and covering epithelium. It is highly vascularized hence they appear red.

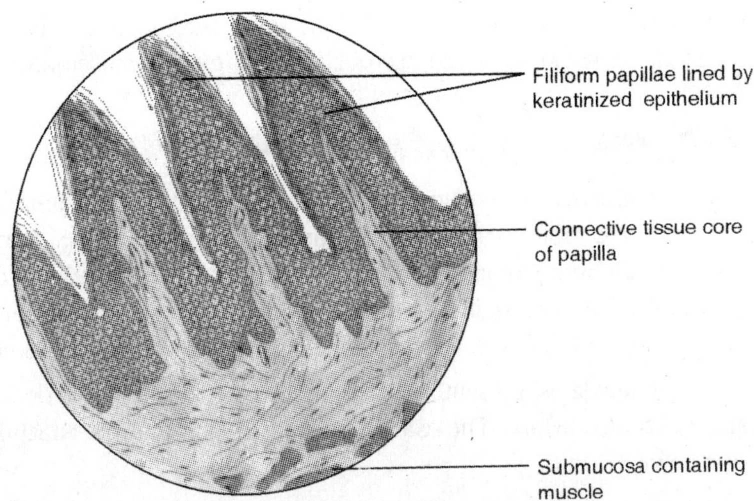

Fig. 9.6: Filiform papillae of tongue (Ref. Fig.10.6–Maji Jose)

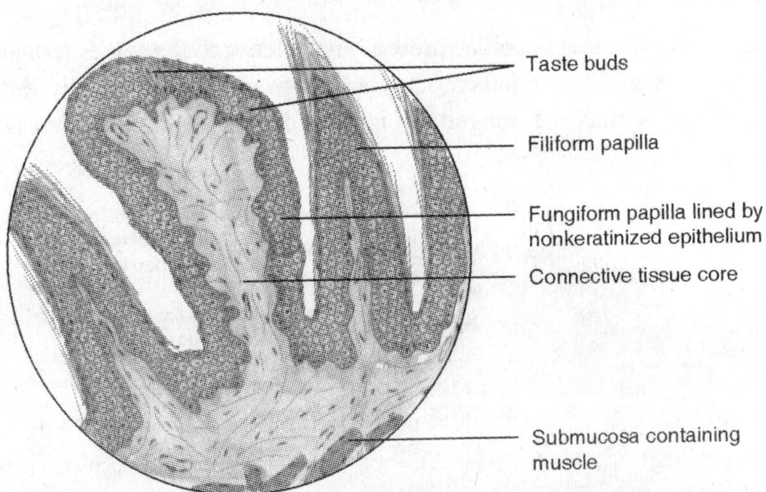

Fig. 9.7: Fungiform papillae of tongue (Ref. Fig.10.8–Maji Jose)

Taste buds

These are small avoid barrel shaped intraepithelial organs that extend from basal lamina to surface of the epithelium. Outer surface taste bud is covered by few flat epithelial cells, which surround a small opening, taste pore Rich plexus of nerves are found below the taste buds.

Lamina propria is dense tissue consisting collagenous fibers and few elastic fibers also contain minor salivary gland, rich innervations especially near taste buds. There is no distinct layer (submucosa) mucosa is bound to the connective tissue surrounding the tongue musculture.

S.Q.A.1 Write briefly about epithelial attachment?

Ans. It is biological mechanism uniting the epithelial cells of the junctional epithelium to the tooth surface via hemidesmosomes and a basal lamina. Junctional epithelium provides the actual attachment of the epithelium to the tooth tissue. The morphologic component of this attachment are basal lamina consisting of both lamina lucida lamina densa and the hemidesmosome.

Lamina lucida is present towards epithelium and lamina densa is towards the tooth surface. The exact biochemical nature of the attachment is not known.

S.Q.A.2 Circumvallate papillae

Ans. These a large papillae present just anterior to the sulcus termanalis. They are 8 to 12 in number. They are large circular and rarely develop above the surface of tongue. It is bounded by a circular furrow.

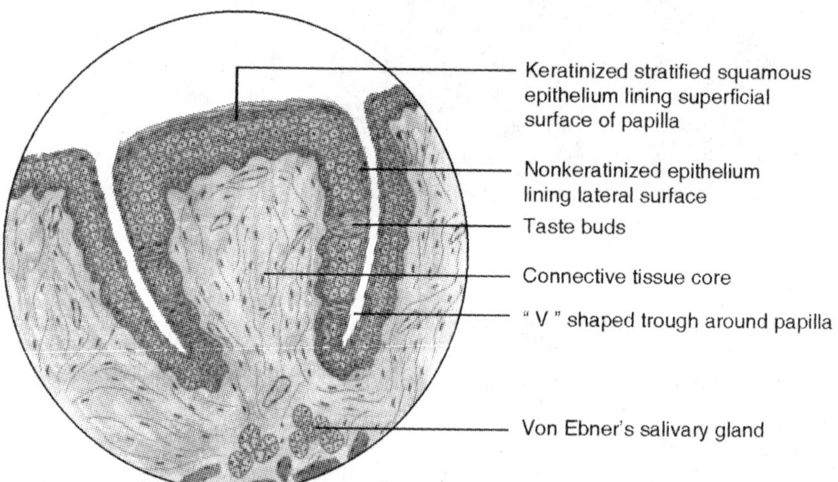

Fig. 9.8 Cirumvallate papilla of tongue (Ref. Fig.10.7–Maji Jose)

Microscopically: Each papilla has central core of connective tissue covered by keratinized epithelium on the lateral surface they contain numerous taste buds. Associated with each papilla are some serous gland called von Ember glands and their duct open in the forrow around papilla.

S.Q.A.3 Non keratinocytes

Ans. These are the cells that are present in oral epithelium other than those forms keratin. These cells include pigment forming melanocytes present in basal layer. Tactile sensory cells called market cells present in basal layer.

Inflammatory associated cells–lymphocyte Langerhans cells–present in suprabasal layer.

S.Q.A.4 Kerationocytes

Ans. Kerationcytes are the basic cells of the oral epithelium and are so named because of its content keratin filament. These keratin filament help in distinguishing them from other cells that non- keratinocytes. Keratinocytes increases in volume in each successive layer from the basal to granular layer.

S.Q.A.5 Alveolar mucosa

Ans. It is a type of lining mucosa that covers the alveolar process and is loosely attached. It is non keratinized with thin epithelium. Lamina propria shows short papilla and contain elastic fibers. Submucosa is loose connective tissue that attached the mucosa to the underlying periosteum covering the alveolar bone.

S.Q.A.6 Gingival Col

Ans. Facial and lingual corner of the interdental gingiva is high with a central valley like area. This central concave area conforming the contact area is called col. The col is lined by a thin nonkeratinized epithelium and it has been suggested that col in most vulnerable to periodontal disease.

S.Q.A.7 Melanocytes

Ans. Are non-keratinocytes present in the basal layer of oral epithelium. These cells are derived embyologically from neural crest cells. Melanocytes lack desmosomes and tonofilaments but posses long dentritic processes that extends into the several layers of keratinocytes

Function: Synthesis of melanin pigment

S.Q.A.8 Papilla of tongue

Ans. The mucous membrane of anterior 2/3rd of tongue have numerous projections called papilla of distinctive appearance. They are present on the dorsal surface of anterior 2/3rd of tongue.

Cirurmvalate papillae: 8 to 12 in number present just anterior to sulcus terminalis

Filliform papillae: They are numerous and are scattered through out the dorsal surface

Fungiform papillae: They are scattered singly among the filiform papillae in the tip of tongue

S.Q.A.9 Dento–gingival junction

Ans. It is a unique anatomic feature concerned with the attachment of the gingiva to the tooth. The gingiva is considered to consist of two part.

1. Masticatory mucosa faces the oral cavity
2. Dentogingival junction which faces the tooth. This is the functional part of periodontium.

The epithelial component of junction is consist of two parts.

- Sulcular epithelium extension of oral epithelium
- Junctional epithelium–derived form dental epithelium and is in contact with tooth

The actual attachment of this by the basal lamina and hemidesmosomes.

S.Q.A.10 Langerhans cells

Ans. These non keratinocytes present in suprabasal layer of oral epithelium. These are dendritic cells, lacks desmosome and tonofilaments. Ultrastructurally, cell is characterized by presence of small rod or flask shaped granule called Birbeck granule. The source of cells in probably the bone narrow.

They have an immunologic function namely recognizing and processing antigenic material.

10

Salivary Glands

L.Q.A.1 Describe difference between serous and mucosa acini?

Ans.

Serous acini	Mucous acini
• Serous acini cells are specialized for the synthesis of storage and secretion of protelin.	• Cells of mucous acini are specialized for the synthesis storage and secretion of their secretory product.
• Typical serous cells are pyromidal shaped, with broad base resting in a thin basal lanima and narrow apex bording the lumen	• Cells are pyramidal in shape with apex towards the lumen. Apical portion of cell appers clear.
• Spherical nucleus and thin rim of cytoplasm is compressed against the base of the cell occassionally binucleated.	• Nucleus is flat oval and is situated at the base.
• It has golgi complex situated either apically or laterally to nucleus.	• It contains more prominent Golgi complex which reflect cells increased carboydrate metabolism.
• Atypical cytoplasm is filled with secretary granules.	• Other cell organelles are least conspicuous are mainly confined to the base of cytoplasm contain scattered cytoplasm secretory droplets.
• Interdigitatrin between the adjacent cells are more.	• Interdigitation between the adjacent mucous cells are less.
• Secretory granules contain protein. After the complex interaction of RE with Golgi, the content of RE is move	• Golgi apparatins play important role in the formation of secretory product because of its high carbohydrate content.

toward trans face of golgi, where they packed into vacoules and finally forms secretory granules.

- Secretion or discharge of the granule, content occurs by a process called exocytosis.
- Secretion of mucous droplet occurs by a somewhat different mechanism than the exocytotic process.

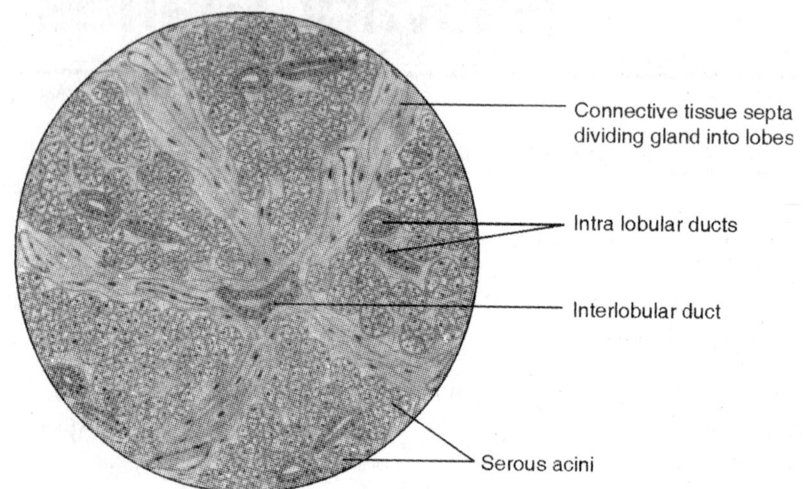

Fig. 10.1: Serous salivary gland (Ref. Fig.11.1–Maji Jose)

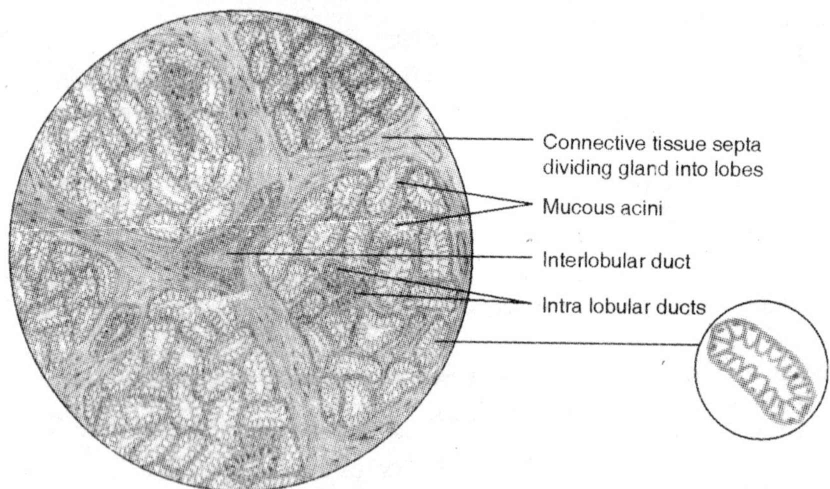

Fig. 10.2: Mucous salivary gland (Ref. Fig.11.2–Maji Jose)

L.Q.A.2 Describe briefly about ductal system of salivary gland

Ans. Ductul system of salivary gland are comprises of varied network of duct progressing from smaller to larger caliber ducts. These are as follows.

Intercalated ⟶ Striated ⟶ Terminal excretory

Ductal system actively participates in the production and modulation of saliva.

(i) **Intercalated duct:** These are the smallest ducts. They are thin branching tubules of varying length that connect the terminal secretory unit to the next larger duct.

Histology: These ducts are lined by a short cuboidal cells with a centrally placed nucleus with little cytoplasm containing some Golgi complex. Secretory granules may sometimes found. Especially in the cells which are close to secretory end piece. These cells have a few microvilli projecting into the lumen of duct.

Adjacent cells are joined apically by junctional complexes and several desmosomes.

Function: Not clearly understood. They are prominent in glands that have watery secretion e.g. parotid gland.

(ii) **Striated duct:** This is in continuation with the intercalated duct but have larger diameter.

Histology: Striated duct is lined by tall columnar cell with large centrally placed nucleus. The most characteristics feature of these cells are prominent striations of plasma membrane (infolding). These striation may extend beyond the lateral border and interdigit with the similar folding of adjacent cells. Large prominent mitochondria arranged along the long axis of the infolds. Apical cytoplasm often contains few scattered vesicles. Few small Golgi complexes and short RER cisternae are found in perinuclear cytoplasm. Lumenal border of cells shows short stubby microvilli. Adjacent cells are joined by junctional complexes and desmosomal attachment.

Function: Modify the secretion passing through the striated duct.

(iii) Terminal Excretory duct: The terminal part of the ductal system of salivary glands in called terminal excretory duct, which ultimately excrete the secretion passing through it into oral cavity.

Histology: It varies as they passes from the striated duct to the oral cavity. Near the striated duct, it is lined by pseudostratified epithelium consisting of tall columnar cells much like the striated cells. As it proceed towards oral cavity the epithelium changes.

Gradually to true stratified epithelium that merges with similar epithelium of oral cavity.

Function: Modify the final saliva by altering the electrolyte concentration and also by adding mucoid component.

L.Q.A.3 Classify salivary glands and describe histological appearance of parotid gland

Ans. Classification

(i) **According to the size and location**

(a) ***Major salivary gland***

- Parotid gland
- Submandibular gland
- Sublingual gland

(b) ***Minor salivary gland***

- Labial and buccal glands
- Glossopalatine glands
- Palatine glands
- Lingual glands

(ii) **According to the nature of their secretion**

- Serous secretory glands
- Mucoid secretory glands

PAROTID GLAND

Parotid gland is the largest of all the salivary glands. It is situated below the external acoustic meatus, between the ramus and stenomastoid. It is a serous type of salivary gland.

Histology

The parotid gland histologically shows following structure.

- Terminal secretory unit
- Ductal system
- Connective tissue elements

Terminal secretory unit

The parotid gland is a pure serous gland and hence the terminal secretory cells are primarily serous cells.

These cells are pyramidal with apex towards the lumen. Nucleus is situated basally. Cytoplasmic organelles present in the cells are functionally related to the protein synthesis. Such as rough endoplasmic–reticulum, Golgi apparatus, R.E.R are large in number. It has large number of secretory granules present in the atypical cytoplasm. Serous cells are surrounded by special type of cells called myoepithelial cell. These cells have a contractile function helps in expeling secretion in the lumen of secretory unit.

Ductal system

Intercalated ducts in porotid glands are numerous and elongated. They are interposed between seromucous acini. It is lined by cuboidal cells. Striated duct are lined by tall columnar cells.

Connective tissue element

Connective tissue of salivary gland is same that of any other connective Tissue, consist of fibroblast, macrophage, mast cells, adipose tissue and plasma cells. Extracellular matix contain collagen fibers and ground substance connective tissue septa between acini have numerous fat cells.

L.Q.A.4 Write about functions of saliva

Ans. Functions of saliva are

1. **Protective**

   Lubricant: glycoprotein content of the saliva makes it mucinous, protect the lining mucosa by forming barrier against noxious stimuli microbial toxins.

Washing action: Flushes away nonadherent bacterial and acellular debris from the mouth.

2. **Buffering:** Saliva has buffering capacity Buffering action is due to the presence of bicarbonates and phosphate.

   Thereby it protects the oral cavity in two way.

   Maintaining PH unsuitable for many bacterial colonization

   Neutralizing acid that are produced by various plaque micro organisms.

3. **Digestion:** Saliva is important for digestion and it has following function.

   Form bolus:

   It contains two enzymes which helps in digestion

   Ptylin or salivary amylase–starch digestion

   Salivary lipase–acts on Triglyceride

   Dilute gastric chyme

4. **Taste:** Saliva dissolves the substances to be tasted and carry them to the taste buds. It contain protein called gusten that is required for growth and maturation of taste buds.

5. **Antimicrobial:** Glycoprotein present forms barrier against microorganism

   Lysozyme has antibacterial effect:

   Antibodies (lgA) agglutinate microorganisms

6. **Maintenance of tooth integrity**

   Saliva is saturated with calcium and phosphate ions. These ions are exchanged with tooth and thereby maintaining the intigrity of tooth. This is important for post eruptive maturation and for repair.

S.Q.A.1 Write briefly about sub-lingual salivary gland.

Ans. It is a smallest of all salivary glands. It is almond shaped. It lies in the floor of mouth between mylohyoid muscle and mucosa of floor of mouth. It is composed of one main gland and several smaller glands. The main duct of gland is called Bartholins duct that opens with or near the submandibular duct. It is a mixed typed of gland.

Histology

As it is a mixed type of salivary gland it consist both serous acini and mucosa acini but mucus secretory units predominate the serous secretory unit. Mucus cells are usually arranged in tubular pattern, serous demilunes may be present at the blind ends of tubules serous acini, are rare.

Intercalated duct are short or may absent, even striated duct are short and are difficult to find. It these the mucous tubules directly opens into duct lined by cuboidal or columnar cells.

S.Q.A.2 Describe the composition of saliva.

Ans.

Composition

Saliva is a watery secretion with pH of about 6.0 to 7.4

- Water content of saliva is about 90% or more of its total volume
- Remaining 1% consists of organic, inorganic and solid.

Inorganic constituents of saliva

Sodium potassium chloride, and bicarbonates, calcium and phosphate.

Organic constituents of siliva

- ***Enzymes:*** Amylase, lipase, proteases orxidases. Lysozyme
- ***Proteins:*** Globulin (IgA) mucin
- ***Carbohydrate:*** rich glycoproteins

S.Q.A.3 Classify oral mucosa and write about specialized mucosa

Ans. Classification of oral mucosa on functional criteria

- Masticatory mucosa – Gingiva, Hard palate
- Lining/reflecting mucosa – Lip, cheek, vestibular fornix, alveolar mucosa, floor of mouth, and soft palate.
- Specialized mucosa – Dorsum of the tongue

Specialized mucosa

It is that part of oral mucosa that cover the dorsum of the tongue. It is highly extensible lining even though it is lining the functionally masticatory area in addition it has different types of lingual papillae. Some of these have mechanical function, and some bears taste buds.

Different types of papillae present are:

- Circumvalate papilla
- Filiform papilla
- Fungiform papilla

S.Q.A.4 Mucous acini

Ans. This is a type of secretory end piece that predominantly consist of mucus cells, They are arranged is various pattern from simple circular to tubular.

The mucus cells are pyramidal in shape with apex towards lumen, nucleus is flat situated towards base. Rough endoplasmic reticulum and few golgi apparatus are found in perinuclear cytoplasm. Cytoplasm near apex appears clear with few secretory droplets.

S.Q.A.5 Myoepithelial cells

Ans. Special type of cells are closely related to the secretory and intercalated duct cells, lying between the basal lamina and basal membrane. Body of cells is small flat nucleus and have numerous branching cytoplasmic processes radiate out. These cells are also called basket cells.

Myoepithelial cells are considered to have contractile function, helping to expel secretions from the lumen of secretory units and ducts.

S.Q.A.6 Ducts of salivary gland

Ans. The duct system of salivary gland is formed by the confluence of small ducts progressing to large caliber ducts.

Intercalated duct ⟶ Striated duct ⟶ Terminal excretory duct.

Intercalated duct

Intercalated duct are the smallest duct within the lobule that connects the secretory unit to striated duct. Intercalated duct are lined by cuboidal cells.

Striated ducts

It is in continuation with the intercalated duct. It is lined by tall columnar cells.Function: modify the secretion passing through it.

Terminal excretory duct

It is terminal part of ductal system that ultimately excreate the secretion in to oral cavity Function: Modify saliva by altering its electrolyte concentration

S.Q.A.7 Minor salivary glands

Ans. The minor salivary glands are located between the epithelium in almost all parts of the oral cavity. These glands usually consist of several small groups of secretory units. Opening via short ducts directly into the mouth.

The minor salivary glands are

- Labial and buccal glands
- Glossopalatine glands
- Palatine glands
- Lingual glands

S.Q.A.8 Von ebner glands

Ans. These are the pure serous gland located between the muscle fibers of the tongue below the circumyallate papillae.

Their ducts opens in the trough around the papillae.

S.Q.A.9 Salivary lipase

Ans. Salivary lipase are secreted by theUon Ebner's gland. Lipase act optimally in acidic pH and acts on the triglycerides, hydrolyzing it. It is a 1st triglyceride hydrolysing enzyme in GIT and act with in stomach.

NOTES

11

Tooth Eruption

L.Q.A.1 Describe tooth eruption

Ans. Tooth eruption is the axial movement of tooth from its developmental position in the jaw to its final position in the oral cavity. Tooth eruption comprises of following physiological tooth movement.

(a) **Pre eruptive tooth movement:** It is a movement of the tooth germ from where it differentrate to the place from where they will erupt. There is sufficient space which is used by the rapid growth of the tooth germs. Both decidous and permanent teeth have this movement.

All these movement occurs in association with growth of jaws

Histology: These movement requires the remodeling of the bony wall around the tooth germ (crypt). This is achieved by selective deposition and resorption of bone, which is carried out by osteoblast and osteoclast respectively.

(b) **Eruptive tooth movement:** During this phase the tooth moves from its position in the jaw where it develops to its functional position in occlusion. The principal direction of this movement is axial.

Histology: During this movement following changes are associated.

(i) Formation of root

(ii) Formation of PDL

(iii) Formation of dentogingival junction

Root formation is initiated by the growth of Hertwigs epithelial sheath. It initiate the differentiation of odontoblast which lay down dentin. With the beginning of root formation many structural changes occurs in the PDL, which is responsible for tooth movement

Significant changes occurs in the tissue overlying the erupting teeth. Resorption of overlying bone once the overlying bone is removed. There is a loss of intervening connective tissue. All this happens due to the following pressure from the erupting tooth cause local Ischemia and necrosis. Also thought the reduced enamel epithelium covering the newly erupting tooth produces certain enzyme which are responsible for such changes that occur. The reduced enamel epithelium and oral epithelium that came in contact starts proliferating to form a solid plug degenerates forming a canal lined by epithelium.

(c) **Post eruptive phase:** Post eruptive moment are those that

(i) Maintain the position of erupted tooth while the jaw continue to grow.

(ii) Compensate the occlusal and proximal wear.These movement continue throughout the life to compensate occlusal and proximal wear.

Histology: It is assumed that continues deposition of cementum around the apices of root. Proximal wear results in mesial or proximal drift. Histologically these drift is seen as selective deposition and resorption of bone on socket wall.

S.Q.A.1 Mechanism of tooth eruption

Ans. Number of theories has been put forward to explain the mechanism of the tooth eruption.

(*a*) **Bone remodeling theory:** Selective resorption and deposition of bone in the socket brings the tooth movement (Eruption)

(*b*) **Root growth theory:** Apical growth of roots results in the axially directed force that bring the eruption

(*c*) **Blood pressure theory:** According to this theory, the tissue around the developing end of root is highly vascular. This vascular pressure is believed to caused axial movement of teeth.

(*d*) **Periodontal ligament traction theory:** It states that the PDL is rich in fibroblasts that contain contractile element. The contraction of these element results in axial movement of the tooth.

(*e*) **Hammock ligament:** A band of fibrous tissue exists below the root apex spanning from one side of the alveolar wall to the other. This fibrous tissue appears to form a network below the developing root and is rich in fluid droplet.

S.Q.A.2 Eruption dates of decidous and permanent teeth

Ans.

(a) **Primary dentition**

	Maxillary	**Mandibular**
Central incisor	71/2 months	6 months
Lateral incisor	19 months	7 months
Canine incisor	18 months	16 months
First molar	14 months	12 months
Second molar	24 months	20 months

(b) **Permanent dentition**

	Maxillary	**Mandibular**
Central incisor	7-8 yrs	6-7 yrs
Lateral incisor	8-9 yrs	7-8 yrs
Canine incisor	11-12 yrs	9-10 yrs
First premolar	10-12 yrs	10-12 yrs
Second premolar	10-12 yrs	11-12 yes
First molar	6-7 yrs	6-7 yrs
Second molar	12-13 yrs	11-13 yrs
Third molar	17-21 yrs	17 –21 yrs

S.Q.A.3 Sequences of maxillary teeth eruption

Ans. The eruption sequence of the permanent dentition may exhibit variation. The frequently seen sequence in the maxillary arch are

6-1-2-4-3-5-7

OR 6-1-2-3-4-5-7

Where as decidous dentition A-B-D-C-E

NOTES

12

Shedding of Decidous Teeth

L.Q.A.1 Write briefly about shedding of decidous teeth

Ans. The physiologic process resulting in the elimination of decidous dentition is called shedding or exfoliation.

Pattern of shedding

The shedding of decidous teeth is the result of progressive resorption of the roots of decidous teeth. Generally the pressure excerted by the growing and erupting permanent tooth dictate the pattern of decidous tooth resoption. Permanent incisor and canine tooth germs develops and move in occlusal and vestibular direction hence the root resorption of decidous incisors and canine begins on their lingual surface. Resorption in the decidous molars begin in the inner aspect because the bicuspids develop in between the roots of decidous.

Histology of shedding

The cells responsible for the remoral of dental hard tissue are called odontoclast. These cells are identical to osteoclast.

Odontoblasts are readily identifiable in light microscope as large multinucleated cell occupying resorption bays on the surface of a dental hard tissue. Cytoplasm is vacuolated and the surface of the cell adjacent to the resorbing hard tissue are ruffled. Odontoclasts are able to resorb all the dental hard tissues including on occasions enamel.

Origin of odontoclast is similar as that of osteoclast. Odontoblasts are most commonly found on root surfaces of the roots in relation to the advancing permanent tooth.

The process of tooth resoption is not continuous since there are periods of rests and repair, however resoption predominates over repair. Repair is achieved by cells resembling cementoblast that lay down collagenous matix

Mechanism of resoption and shedding

Mechanism is not truely understood. It seems that pressure from the erupting succesional tooth plays key role because of odontoclasts appear at predicted sites of pressure. The odontoclasts attaches to the dental hard tissue and secret their enzymatic contents into the microenvironment and degrade organic matix.

S.Q.A.1 Odontoclasts

Ans. Odontoclasts are (elastic) or resorptive cells that have ability to remove all dental hard tissue. These cells are identical to osteoclast. Odontoclasts are large multinucleated that occupies the resorptive bays on root surface. Border of cell facing towards the resorption surface of root is ruffled. Cytoplasm near the ruffled border is clear and devoid of organelles but rich in filaments. Origin of odontoclast is similar to that of osteoclast.

NOTES

13 Temporomandibular Joint

S.Q.A.1 Enumerate the ligaments of TMJ and their function

Ans. Ligaments that are associated with the TMJ are

- Lateral or Temporomandibular ligament
- Sphenomandibular ligament
- Stylomandibular ligament

The only important function of these ligament is to provide stability to the joint. Among three ligaments, temporomandibular ligament has any functional significance and other two have only casual relation with TMJ.

NOTES

NOTES

14

Maxillary Sinus

S.Q.A.1 Maxillary sinus

Ans. Also called antrum of Highmore. It is a largest of all paranasal sinus present in the body of maxilla. Pyramidal in shape with base towards the lateral wall of nose and apex directed toward zygomatic process of maxilla. It opens into the middle meatus of nose. Microscopically three distinct layer surrounds the maxillary sinus.

- Epithelial layer
- Basal lamina
- Subepithelial layer

Epithelium: Pseudostratified, columnar and ciliated, derived from olfactory epithelium

S.Q.A.2 Functions of Maxillary sinus

Ans. Little known about the function of paralnasal sinus

- Humidification and warming of inspired air
- Resonance to the voice
- Lightening of skull weight
- Enhancement of faciocranial resistance to mechanical shock
- Production of bacteriocidal lysozymes in nasal cavity

NOTES

Section–2

DENTAL ANATOMY

15

Introduction

L.Q.A.1 Write briefly about tooth numbering system.

Ans.

Human dentition consist of two sets of teeth

(i) Primary/Decidous

(ii) Permanent

Decidous teeth are 20 in number, 10 in each arch. The permanent teeth are 32 in number, 16 in each arch.

DENTAL FORMULAE

Denomination and number is used to express the formula e.g. denomination I for incisor.

Dental formula for decidous teeth

$$I\frac{2}{2} \quad C\frac{1}{1} \quad M\frac{2}{2}$$

Dental formula for permanent teeth

Methods of tooth numbering:

upper right	upper left
lower right	lower left

1. Zigmondy's and palmar method

Oral cavity is divided into four quadrant

By this method the dentition is notated as Decidous dentition

E D C B A	A B C D E
E D C B A	A B C D E

Permanent dentition

8 7 6 5 4 3 2 1	1 2 3 4 5 6 7 8
8 7 6 5 4 3 2 1	1 2 3 4 5 6 7 8

2. Universal method

Using this system the decidous teeth are notated as. In maxillary arch it begins with letter A from right through J whereas in mandibular arch it begin with letter K from left through T.

A B C D E	F G H I J
T S R Q P	O N M L K

Similarly for the permant teeth in maxillary arch it begins with number 1 from right through 16 where as in mandibalar urch it begins with number 17 from left through 32.

1 2 3 4 5 6 7 8	9 10 11 12 13 14 15 16
32 31 30 29 28 27 26 25	24 23 22 21 20 19 18 17

3. FDI system (Two digit system)

In two digit system 1st digit indicates the quadrant e.g.. For permanent dentition 1 to 4 beginning with right quadrant, for decidous dentition 5 to 8 similar to permanent Second digit indicates the tooth.

It is expressed as Decidous dentition:

55 54 53 52 51	61 62 63 64 65
85 84 83 82 81	71 72 73 74 75

Permanent dentition:

18 17 16 15 14 13 12 11	21 22 23 24 25 26 27 28
48 47 46 45 44 43 42 41	31 32 33 34 35 36 37 38

S.Q.A.1 Mamelons

Ans. These are small rounded eminence present on the incisal edges of newly erupted incisors. These are commonly seen in maxillary incisor. They are three in number each representing one lobe. Soon after eruption they are worn down by use unless through malalignment, they excape incisal wear.

S.Q.A.2 Cingulum

Ans. It is a lobe like structure present on the lingual surface of anterior teeth. It makes the bulk of the cervical 3rd of the lingual surface. Its convexity mesiodistally resembles a girdle encircling the lingual surface at the cervical third. In each dentition they are 12 in number

S.Q.A.3 Ridges

Ans. A ridge is any linear elevation on the surface of a tooth and is named according to its location.

(a) **Marginal ridges:** These are rounded borders of the enamel that form the mesial and distal margins of the occlusal surfaces of premolars and molars and the mesial and distal margins of the lingual surfaces of the incisors and canines.

(b) **Triangular ridges:** These descend from the tips of the cusps of molars and premolars toward the central part of the occlusal surfaces. They are so named because the slopes of each side of surfaces. They are so named because the slopes of each side of the ridge are inclined to resemble two sides of a triangle.

(c) **Transverse ridge:** When buccal and lingual triangular ridges join they form transverse ridge. Present on posterior tooth.

(d) **Oblique ridge:** The oblique ridge is a ridge crossing obliquely the occlusal surfaces of maxillary molars. It is formed by the union of the triangular ridge of the distobuccal cusp and the distal ridge of the mesiopalatal cusp.

S.Q.A.4 Pits

Ans. Are the small pin point depression located at the junction of developmental groves or are the terminals of those grooves. E.g.-central pit, is a term used to describe a landmark in the central fossa of molars where developmental grooves join.

S.Q.A.5 Fossa

Ans. A fossa is an irregular depression or concavity.

1. **Lingual fossa-** Present on the lingual surface of incisors.
2. **Central fossa-** Present on the occlusal surface of molars. They are formed by the converging of ridges terminating at a central point in the botton of the depression, where there is a junction of grooves.
3. **Triangular fossa-** They are found on molars and premolars on the occlusal surfaces mesial or distal to marginal ridges. They are sometimes found on lingual surfaces of maxillary incisors at the edge of the lingual fossa where the marginal ridges and the cingulum meet.

S.Q.A.6 Crown

Ans. Crown is that part of tooth that above the CEJ Crown is described in two ways.

Anatomical crown: part of tooth that is covered by cementum.

Clinical crown: part of tooth that exposed to oral cavity.

Crown may be divided into thirds in 3 directions, incisocervically or occlusocervically, mesiodistally labiolingually or buccolingually Mesiodistally: Mesial, Middle and distal 3rd. labio or buccolingually: Labial/buccal, Middle and lingual. Occluso-or incisocervically:Incisal/ occlusal, middle and cervical

S.Q.A.7 Line angles

Ans. Is formed by the junction of two surfaces. It derive its name from the combination of the two surfaces: that join.

1. **Line angles of anterior teeth**

   Mesiolabial

   Distolabial

   Mesiolingual

   Distolingual

   Labioincisal

   Linguoincisal

   Because the mesial and distal incisal angles of anterior teeth are and rounded, mesioincisal line angles and distoincisal line angles are usually considered nonexistent. They are spoken of as mesial and distal incisal angles only.

2. **Line angles of posterior teeth**

   Mesioocclusal

   Mesolingual

   Buccoocclusal

   Lingocclusal

   Distolingual

   Distobuccal

   Mesiobuccal

   Distoocclusa

S.Q.A.8 Point angles

Ans.

Point angles are formed by the junction of three surfaces.Point angles derives its name from the combination of the names of surfaces forming it

Point angles of anterior teeth

- Mesiolabioincisal

- Distolabioincisal
- Mesiolinguoincisal
- Distolinguoincisal

Point angles of posterior teeth

- Mesiobuccooclusal
- Distobuccoocclusal
- Mesiolinguoocclusal
- Distolinguoocclusal

NOTES

16

The Primary Teeth

L.Q.A.1 Describe in detail about the difference between the permanent and decidous dentition

Ans.

Permanent teeth	Primary teeth
• 32 in number, 16 in each arch	• Primary teeth are 20 in number, 10 in each arch
• Cervicoincisal dimension is greater than mesiodistal dimension	• Crown of primary teeth are wider mesodisatally than the cervicoincisally
• They do not have any marked cervical ridge.	• Have prominent cervical ridge. cervical on buccal surface
• Do not have such constrictions.	• It shows marked cervical constriction
• Root are bulky	• Root are narrow and thin
• No flared roots	• Flared roots
• Pulp chambers are small and pulp horns are at lower level as compaired to primary	• Pulp chambers are large in size with higher pulp horns
• It appears yellowish in color because of thicker and more translucent enamel	• Primary teeth appears lighter in color because of thin enamel.
• Occlusal table is broad as compaired to primary.	• Occlusal table is narrow

NOTES

17 General Consideration in the Physiology of the Permanent Dentition

S.Q.A.1 Curve of spee

Ans. It refers to the antero posterior curvature of the occlusal surfaces. Begins at the tip of the lower cuspid and following the cusp tips of the biuspids and molars continue as an arc through the condyle. Curve results from the variation in axial alingment of the lower teeth.

S.Q.A.2 Elevation of surface of crown

Ans. Various elevated structures are present on the surface of crown.

Cusp: Elevation on the crown portion of a tooth making up a divisional part of the occlusal surface.

Tuburcle: Smaller elevation on some portion of crown produce an extra formation of enamel.

Cingulum: Is a lingual lobe of an interior tooth makes bulk of cervical 3rd of lingual surface

Ridge: Are linear elevation e.g. buccal incisal marginal ridge found on occlusal surface at margins and distal margins of premolar and molars.

Oblique ridge: Is a ridge crossing obliquely the occlusal surface of maxillary molars.

S.Q.A.3 Embrassures

Ans. It is also known as spillways. When the two teeth in the same arch are in the contact then the area adjust the contact point are called embrassures.

When viewed from occlusal surface the area buccal to contact area is called as buccal or labial interproximal embrassure and area lingual to contact area is called as lingual interproximal embrassure.

When viewed from labial side than the area of occlusal side is called as occlusal or incisal embrassure and area cervical to contact area is called as gingival embrassure.

Embrassure serves two purposes

(i) Makes spillway for the escapement of food during mastication

(ii) It prevents the food being forced through the contact area

NOTES

18 Permanent Maxillary and Mandibular Incisors

S.Q.A.1 Measurement and chronology of permanent maxillary central incisor

Ans.

Measurement

Cervicoincisal length of crown	= 10.5 mm
Root length	= 13 mm
Mesiodistal diameter of crown	= 8.5 mm
Mesiodistal diameter of crown at cervix	= 7.0 mm
Labio or buccolingual width of crown	= 7.0 mm
Labio or buccolingual width of crown at cervix	= 6.0 mm
Curvature of cervical line mesially	= 3.5 mm
Curvature of cervical link distally	= 2.5 mm

Chronology

1st evidence of calcification	= 3–4 month
Enamel completed	= 4–5 yrs
Eruption	= 7–8 yrs
Root completed	= 10 yrs

NOTES

19

Permanent Maxillary and Mandibular Canine

L.Q.A.1 Describe in detail chronology and morphology of maxillary permanent canine

Ans. **Chronology of Maxillary permanent canine**

1st evidence of calcification	– 4 to 5 month
Enamel completed	– 6 to 7 years
Eruption	– 11 to12 yrs
Root completed	– 13 to15 yrs

Morphology

Labial view

Form the labial view the mesial half resembles the portion of an incisor where as distal half resembles a portion of premolar

- Mesially the outline of crown may be convex from cervical to the contact point. The contact area on the mesial aspect is at the junction of middle and incisal 3rd of the crown.
- Distally the outline of the crown is usually concave. Between the cervical line and the contact point distal contact area is at the center of middle 3rd of crown.
- Labial surface of the crown is smooth with no developmental lines except shallow depression mesially and distally. In the center of labial surface there is ridge that represent the middle labial lobe.
- Root appears slender. It is conical in form with a blunt apex. In the apical region root have sharp curve either mesially or distally.

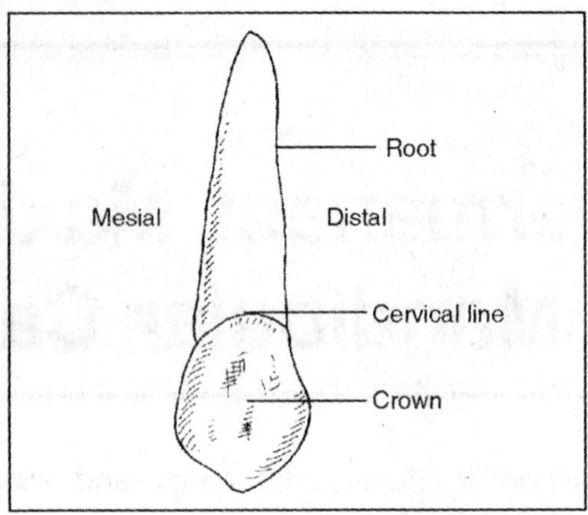

Fig. 19.1: Maxillary left canine, labial aspect

Lingual aspect

From this aspect the crown and root appear narrow. The cingulum is large and in some instances is pointed like a small cusp.

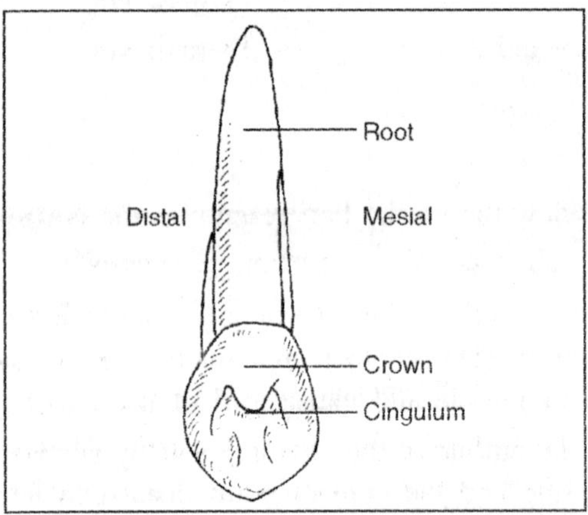

Fig. 19.2: Maxillary left canine, Lingual aspect

- Occasionally a well developed lingual ridge may appear. There may be shallow depression between this ridge and marginal ridges. It these depressions are present than they are called mesial and distal fossae.
- The lingual portion of root is narrow because of this much of mesial and distal surface of the root in visible from this aspect.

Mesial aspect

Mesial aspect of maxillary canine represent the outline form of anterior tooth. It shows greater bulk in labiolingual direction than any other anterior tooth

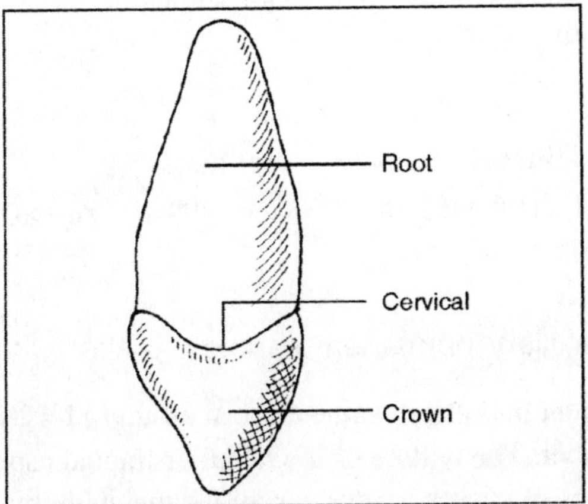

Fig. 19.3: Maxillary left canine, Mesial aspect

- *Labial outline:* exhibit convex from cervical line to cusp tip.
- Lingual outline, convex line describing cingulum this convex line straighten in middle 3rd and again it become convex incisally.
- Root appears conical with a tapered or blunt apex.
- Tip of the cusp in relation to the long axis of root, lies lingually

Distal aspect

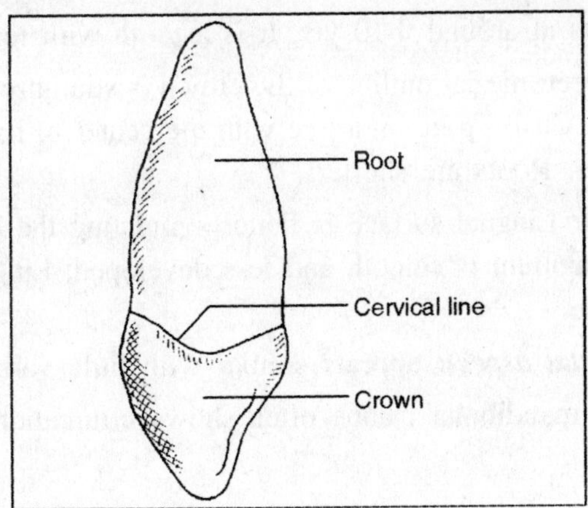

Fig. 19.4: Maxillary left canine, Distal aspect

Some what same as that of mesial aspect, shows little variations. Cervical line exhibit less curvature. Surface display more concavity more pronounced developmental depression on the distal surface of root.

Incisal aspect

Labiolingual dimension is greater than mesiodistal tip. The cusp is labial to the center of crown.

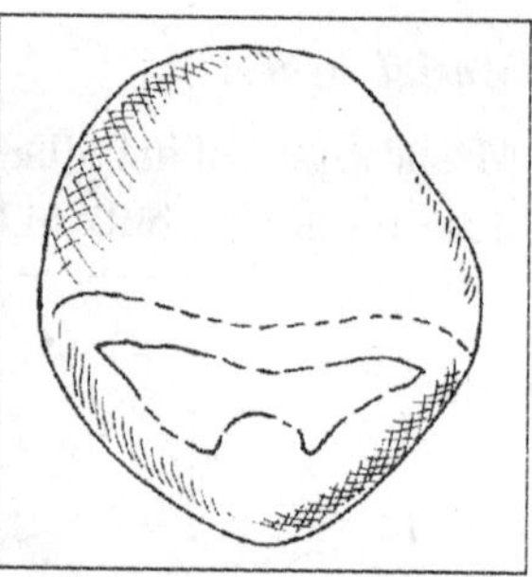

Fig. 20.5: Maxillary left canine, incisal aspect

S.Q.A.1 Maxillary permanent canine

Ans. Permanent maxillary canine erupt at around 11-12 yrs of age. They are two in number. The outline of the labial or lingual aspect of maxillary canine is a series of curves or arcs except for the angle made by the tip of cusp contact points of canine on either side of tooth are in different level.

The labial surface is smooth with a prominent central ridge. Lingual aspect of the crown has a large cingulum. Occasionally, it has lingual ridge dividing the lingual fossa into mesial and distal.

Root: Is slender with blunt apex. Root of maxillary canine is longest of all teeth. Apically it may curve mesially or distally.

S.Q.A.2 Mandibular permanent canine

Ans. It erupts at around 9-10 yrs. It is a tooth with longer crown.

Labial aspect: mesial outline of the crown is straight with the mesial outline of root. Cusp lip lie on a line with the center of root mesial cusp ridge is smaller. Roots are shorter.

Lingual aspect: Lingual surface is flatter simulating the lingual surface of incisors. Cingulum is smooth and less developed. Lingually the root appears narrow.

Mesial and distal aspect: appears similar with little variation.

Root: Root of mandibular canine often shows bifurcation.

20 Permanent Maxillary Premolars

L.Q.A.1 Describe in detail morphology of maxillary 1st premolar

Ans.

Buccal aspect

The tooth resembles canine and roughly trapezoidal in shape.

- Mesial outline of the crown is slightly concave from cervical line to contact point
- Distal outline appears straight below the cervical line
- Both the distal and mesial contact area are broader.
- Buccal surface is convex, showing a well developed buccal ridge.
- Root trunk is long

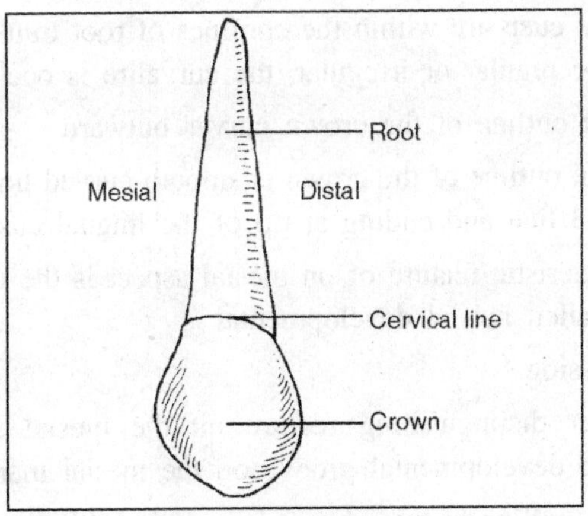

Fig. 20.1: Maxillary left first premolar, buccal aspect

Lingual aspect

Crown tapers towards lingual surface since the lingual cusp is narrower mesiodistally lingual cusp is smooth and spheroidal with pointed cusp lip.

Mesial and distal outline is convex, cervical line is irregular with slight curvature towards the root since the lingual is not so long, buccal cusp in visible from the aspect.

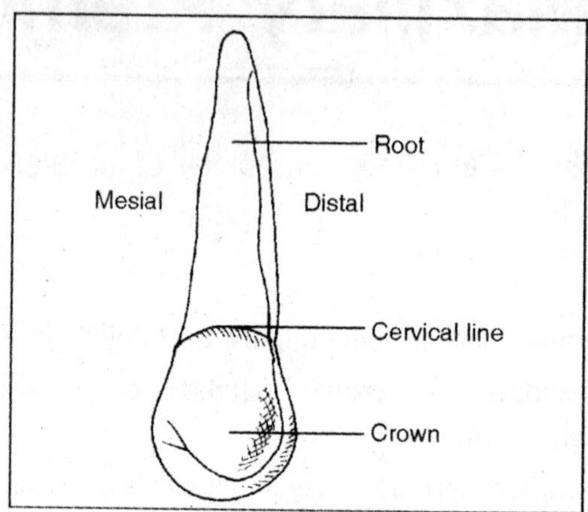

Fig. 20.2: Maxillary left first premolar, lingual aspect

Mesial aspect

Roughly trapezoidal in shape

- Tips of cusp are within the confines of root trunk. Cervical line may be regular or irregular, the curvalire is occlusally
- Buccal outline of the crown curves outward
- Lingual outline of the crown is smooth curved line starting from cervical line and ending at tip of the lingual cusp
- Characteristic feature of on mesial aspect is the marked depression called mesial developmental
- Depression
- Another distinguishing feature on the mesial aspect is well defined developmental groove on the mesial marginal ridge.
- Buccal outline of buceal root is straight with a tendency toward lingual inclination
- Lingual outline of lingual root is also straight but may not exhibit curvature

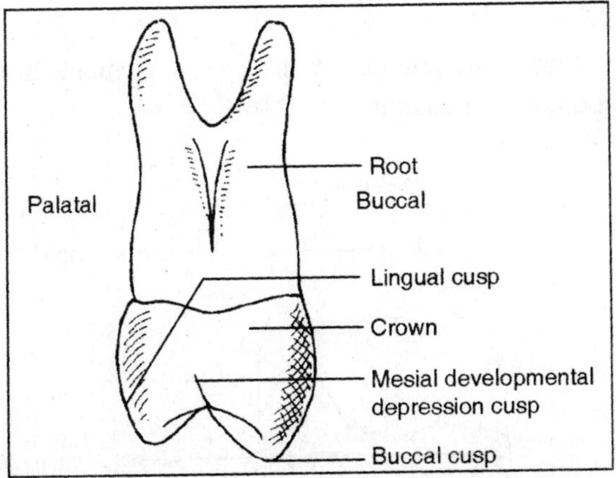

Fig. 20.3: Maxillary left first premolar, mesial aspect

Distal aspect

Almost similar to mesial espect with following difference from the mesial aspect.

- Curvature of cervical line is less.
- No deep developmental grooves on distal marginal ridge.
- Root trunk is flattened on distal surface with no outstanding developmental signs.

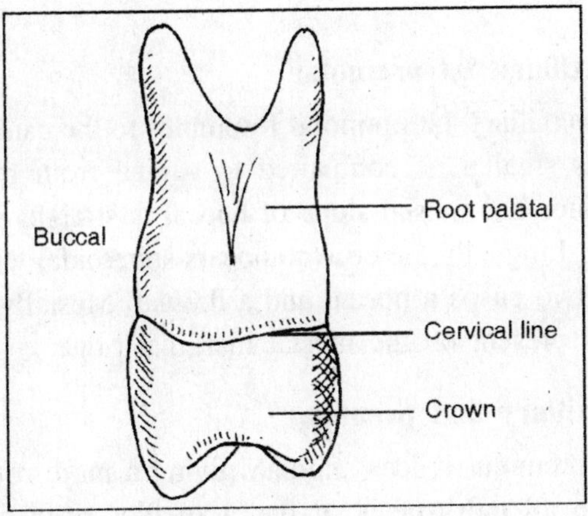

Fig. 20.4: Maxillary left first premolar, distal aspect

Occlusal surface

- Hexagonal in shape which is not equilateral

- Crown is wider on buccal than on lingual
- Buccolingual dimension of the crown is much greater than the mesiodistal dimension.

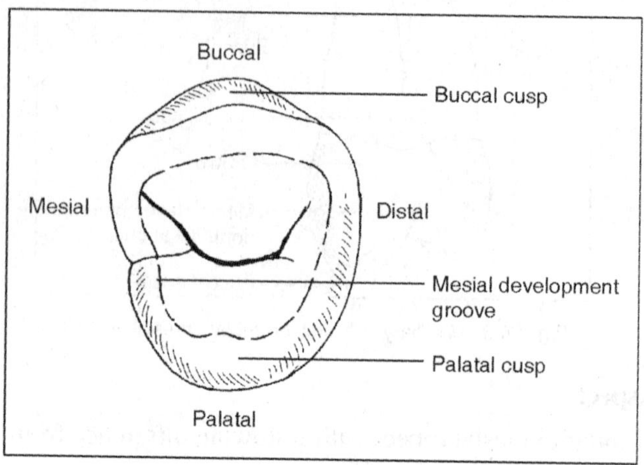

Fig. 21.5: Maxillary left first premolar, occlusal aspect

S.Q.A.1 Crown morphology of maxillary 1st premolar and 2nd premolars

Ans.

Crown of maxillary 1st premolar

The crown of maxillary 1st premolar resembles to the canine from buccal aspect but it is smaller as compaired to canine from buceal expect it appears trapezoid. The mesial slope of buccal is straight and longer than the distal slope. Lingually the crown appears spheroidal with lingual cusp smaller. It has two cusps a buccal and a lingual. Mesially deep development groove is present on the mesial marginal ridge.

Crown of maxillary 2nd premolar

Maxillary 2nd premolar is lees angular, giving a more rounded effect to the crown from all the aspects. It has a smaller cervicoocclusally and also mesiodistally. The two cusps buccal and lingual are of almost same height.

S.Q.A.2 Maxillary 1st premolar

Ans. Maxillary 1st premolar are two in number. Present in either side of each jaw resembling the canine. It develops from 4 lobes.

Buccal aspect: It appears trapezoidal with mesial slope straight and longer than the distal slope. Buccal cusp in long and pointed. Buccal surface shows strong well developed ridge called buccal ridge

Lingual aspect: Lingually appears spherical with lingual cusp smaller as compaired to buccal cusp. Lingual surface show well developed lingual ridge.

Mesial aspect: Roughly trapezoidal tips of cusps are within the confine of root trunk. Buccal outline curves outward below the cervical line. Lingual outline of the crown may be described as a smoothly curved line starting at the cervical line and ending at tip of lingual cusp. A distinguishing point on mesial aspect is well developed mesial developmental depression.

Distal aspect: From this aspect all the features are more or less similar to the mesial aspect. There is no developmental depression on distal aspect. Less curved cervical line on distal than on mesial surface.

Occlusal surface: Roughly hexagonal that is circumscribed by the cusp ridge and marginal ridges. The well defined central developmental groove divides the surface buccolingually

Roots: Most maxillary 1st molars have two roots and two root canals. Buccal and palatal

NOTES

21 Permanent Mandibular Premolars

L.Q.A.1 Describe crown morphology of mandibular 1st premolars.

Ans. Mandibular premolars are four in number two are situated in right side of mandible and two are in left side. The 1st premolars are developed from four lobes where as mandibular 2nd premolars and developed from five lobes.

Mandibular 1st premolar

1st premolar is always smaller of two mandibular premolars. The mandibular 1st premolar has many of characteristics of small canine. The 1st premolar has a large buccal cusp which is long and well formed with a small nonfunctioning lingual cusp.

Buccal aspect

The form of 1st premolar is symmetrical bilaterally, The middle buccal lobe is well developed. The Mesial cusp ridge is shorter than the distal cusp ridge.

The contact areas are broad from this aspect and at same level mesial and distal. Mesial outline of crown is straight or slightly concave above the cervical line to a point where it joins the curvature of the mesial contact area.

Distal outline of the crown is slightly concave above cervical line to a point where it is confluent with the curvature describing the distal contact area. The crest of curvature of the cervical line buccally approaches the center of the root buccally.

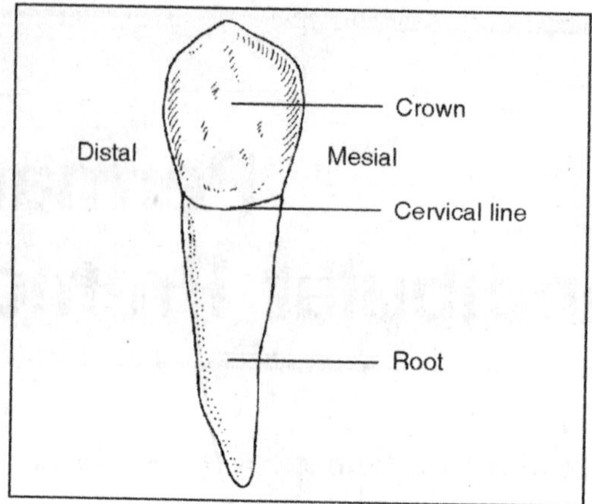

Fig. 21.1: Mandibular right first premolar, buccal aspect

Lingual aspect

The crown of the mandibular 1st premolar tapers towards the lingual, since the lingual measurement is less than that buccally. The lingual cusp in always small. The occlusal surface slopes greatly towards the lingual in cervical direction down to the short lingual cusp. Most of the occlusal surface of this tooth can be seen from this. The cervical portion of the crown lingually is narrow and convex. Although lingual cusp is not developed properly, it is pointed. Characteristic of lingual surface of mandibular 1st premolar is M.L. developmental groove which is a demarcation between the M.B lobe and lingual lobe.

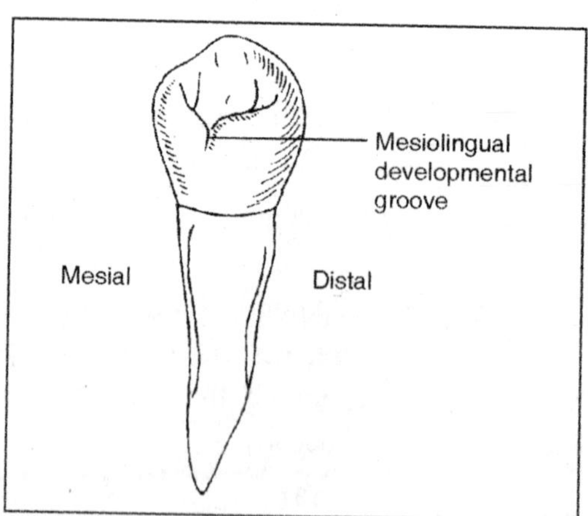

Fig. 21.2: Mandibular right first premolar, lingual aspect

Mesial aspect

Crown outline is roughly rhomboidal and the tip of the buccal cusp is nearly centered over the root. The convexity of the outline of the lingual lobe in lingual to the outline of root. The mandibular 1st premolar when viewed mesially often shows the buccal cusp centred over the root. Buccal outline of the crown from this aspect is prominently curved from the cervical line to the tip of the buccal cusp the crest of the curvature is near the middle third of the crown lingual outline of crown, respresentative of the lingual outline of the lingual cusp is a curved outline of less convexity than that of the buccal surface.

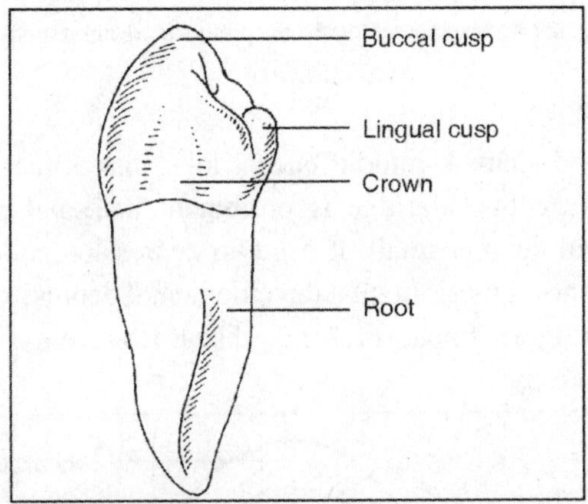

Fig. 21.3: Mandibular right first premolar, mesial aspect

Some of the occlusal surface may be seen from this aspect. The cervical line on the mesial surface is rather regular cerving occlusally. The crest of the curvature is centered buccolingually.

Distal aspect

Distal aspect is more or less similar to that of mesial aspect and differ from mesial aspect in some respects.

- Distal marginal ridge is higher.
- Marginal ridge have no developmental groove.
- Distal contact area is broader.
- Curature of cervical line may be same as that of mesial or less.

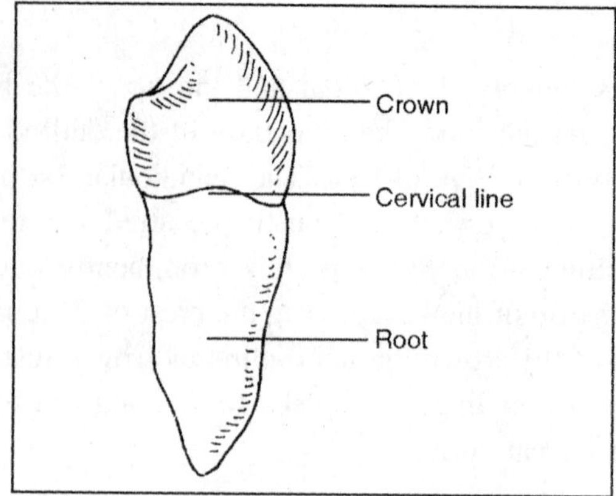

Fig. 21.4: Mandibular right first premolar, distal aspect

Occlusal aspect

Roughly diamond shaped, middle buccal lobe makes the major portion of occlusal surface buccal ridge is prominent marginal ridge are well developed lingual cusp is small. It has two depression called mesial and distal fossae. It shows mesiolingual developmental depression and groove. Mesial fossa is more linear in form, distal fossa may contain distal developmental groove.

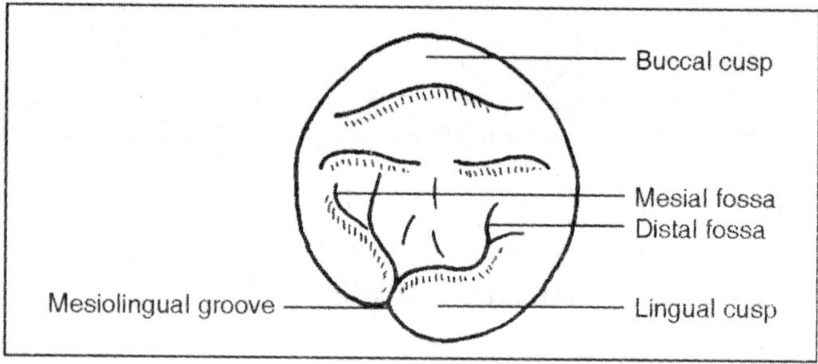

Fig. 21.5: Maxillary left first premolar, occlusal aspect

L.Q.A.2 Describe in detail morphology of mandibular right 2nd premolar

Ans. It develops from five lobes 3 buccal and 2 lingual lobes. The 2nd p. molar have 3 well formed cusps, one large buccal and two small lingual cusps.

Buccal aspect

From buccal aspect the tooth resembles the mandibular 1st premolar with a shorter buccal cusp than 1st premolar. Contact areas are broad both mesial and distal

Root is broader mesiodistally that of 1st premolar.

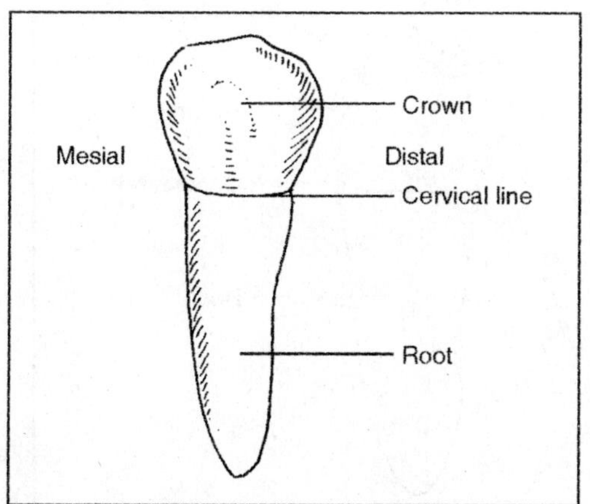

Fig. 21.6: Mandibular left second premolar, buccal aspect

Lingual aspect

Shows considerable variation from that of 1st premolar. Lingual cusps (lobes) are well develops as compaired to that of 1st premolar because of well developed lingual cusps occlusal surface is less visible from this aspect. Lingual aspect is smooth and spheroidal having a bulbous form above the constricted cervical portion

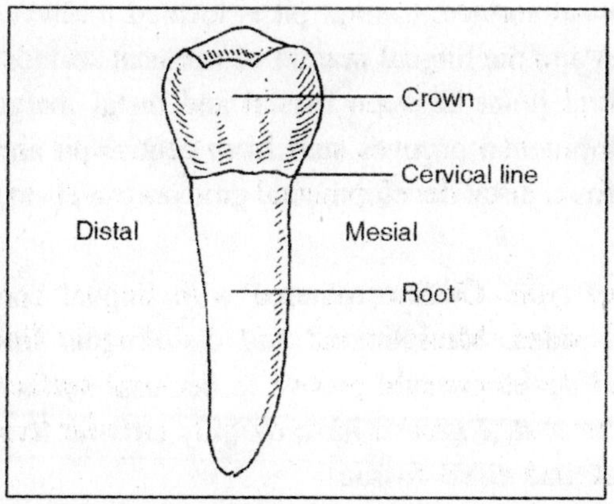

Fig. 22.7: Mandibular left 2nd premolar, lingual aspect

Masial aspect

Crown and root are wider buccalingually. Buccal cusp in not nearly centered over the root and is shorter as compaired to buccal cusp of 1st premolar. Marginal ridges are well developed and at right angle to the long axis of the tooth. There is no developmental groove.

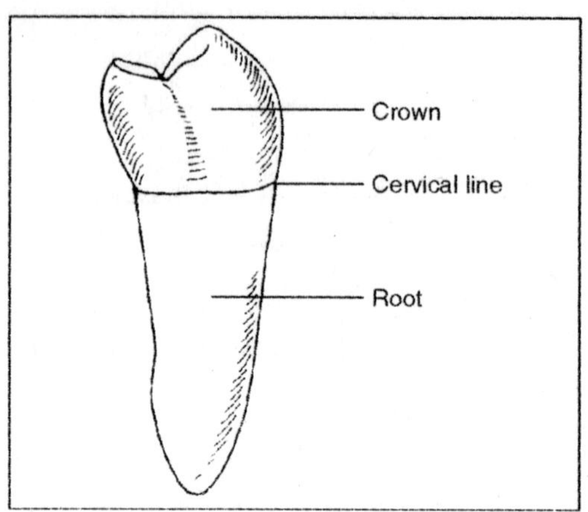

Fig. 22.8: Mandibular left second premolar, mesial aspect

Occlusal aspect

Occlusal surface of tooth shows variation depending open cusp. There cusp types appears: square, lingual to buccal cusp ridges Two cusp type appears: round, lingual to buccal cusp ridges

Each cusp has well formed triangular ridges separated by deep developmental grooves. These grooves convert in a central pit and form a 'Y' on the occlusal surface. Central pit is located midway between the buccal cusp ridges and the lingual margin of occlusal surface and slightly. Distal to the central point between masial and distal marginal ridges.

Mesial developmental grooves start from central pit and ends in the mesial triangular fossa distal developmental grooves travels in a distobuccal direction.

The two cusp type: Outline rounded with lingual convergence of mesial and distal sides. Mesiolingual and distolingual line angles are rounded. A central developmental groove in occlusal surface travels in a M.D direction. The central groove have roughly circular terminal depression called mesial and distal fossae.

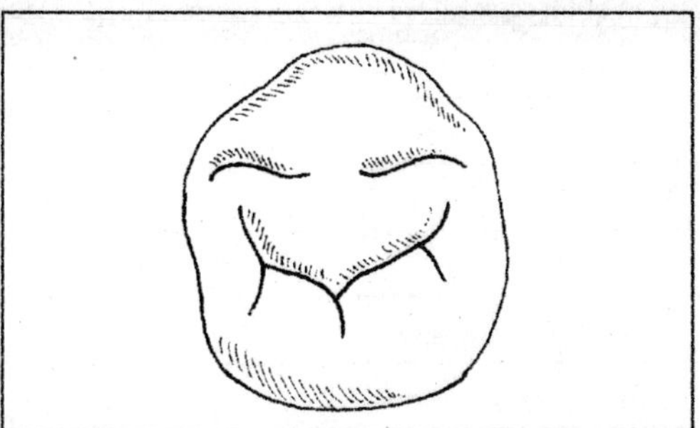

Fig. 22.9: Mandibular left second premolar, occlusal aspect

Distal aspect

Distal aspect is similar to that of mesial aspect, except that the more occlusal surface is seen from this aspect. Distal marginal ridge is at lower level to that of mesial marginal ridge. The crown of tooth is tilted distally to the long axis of the tooth.

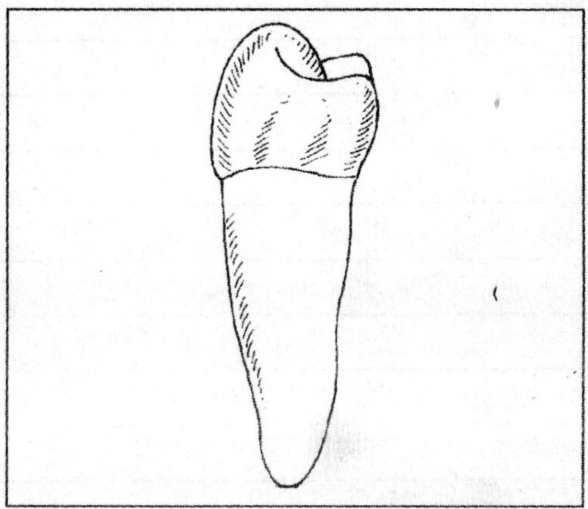

Fig. 22.10: Mandibular left second premolar, distal aspect

NOTES

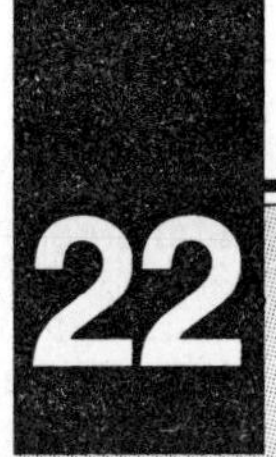

22 Permanent Maxillary Molars

L.Q.A.1 Describe the morphology of maxillary permanent 1st molar

Ans. These are the largest and the strongest maxillary teeth by virtue both of their bulk and their achorage in the jaws. The maxillary first molar have large crown with four well developed cusp two buccal and two lingual cusps. They have 3 roots two buccal and one palatal.

Buccal aspect

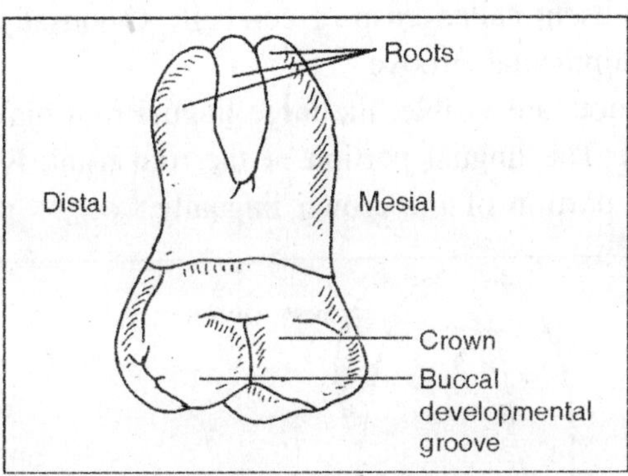

Fig. 22.1: Maxillary right first molar, buccal aspect

The crown is roughly trapezoid from this aspect. All the four cusps are seen mesiobuccal, distobuccal, mesiopalatal and distopalatal. The mesiobuccal cusp is broader than the distobuccul cusp and its mesial slope meets its distal slope at an obtuse angle. Both the buccal cusps are divided by buccal developmental groove. It extends from occlusal surface halfway towards apically and it gradually fades out. The cervical line of the crown does not have much curvature from mesial to distal. The line is geneıally convex with the convexity towards the roots. The mesial outline of the crown from this aspect follows a nearly straight path downwards and mesially curving occlusally as it reaches the crest. The distal outline of crown is convex (spheroidal).

All the 3 roots may be seen from the buccal aspect. The axes of roots are inclined distally. The roots are not straight however the buccal roots showing an indication to curvature half way between the point of bifurcation and the apices. The point of bifurcations of the two buccal roots is located approximately 4mm above cervical line.

Lingual aspect

From the palatal aspect the outline is reverse of buccal aspect. Only the palatal cusps are seen from this aspect [mesiopalatal and distopalatal]. M palatal cusp is much larger, that is about M.D. width of cusp is about three fifth of MD crown diameter. The distopalatal cusp is spheroidal and smooth. Both cusp is divided by a developmental groove called palatal developmental groove. On the lingual surface of mesiopalatal cusp and fifth cusp in present called cusp of cerebelli. Occlusally outlined as an irregular developmental groove.

All three roots are visible, the large lingual root making up most of the foreground. The lingual portion of the root trunk is continues with entire cervical portion of the crown lingually.

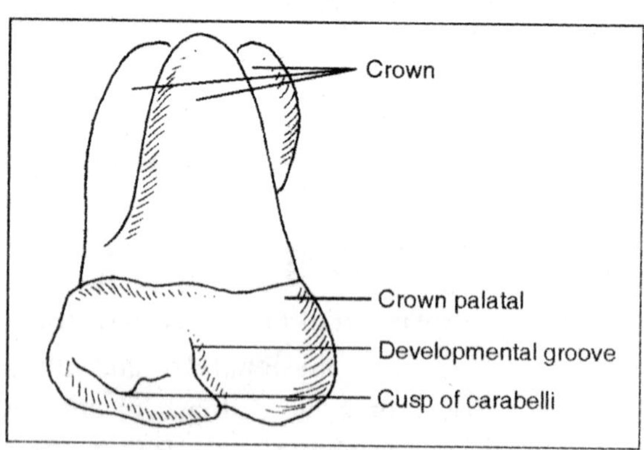

Fig. 22.2: Maxillary right first molar, palatal aspect

Mesial aspect

Form the mesial aspect the buccal outline from cervical line, it starts as arc to its crest, than a shallow concavity followed by slightly convex as if progresses downward and inward to circumseribe the M.D cusp. The palatal outline of crown curves outward and palatally approximately to the same extent as on buccal side except that level of crest of curvature is near the middle 3rd of the crown rather than a point. Fifth cusp is visible. The mesial marginal ridge is irregular. The cervical line is irregular curving occlusally. Mesial contact area is closer to the cervical line approximately at the junction of middle and occlusal 3rd of the crown.

The mesiobuccal root is broad and flattened on its mesial surface. This flattened surface often exhibits smooth flutings for part of its length. Root end is blunt. Level of bifurcation is closer to cervical line Lingual root is longer than the mesial root but is narrower.

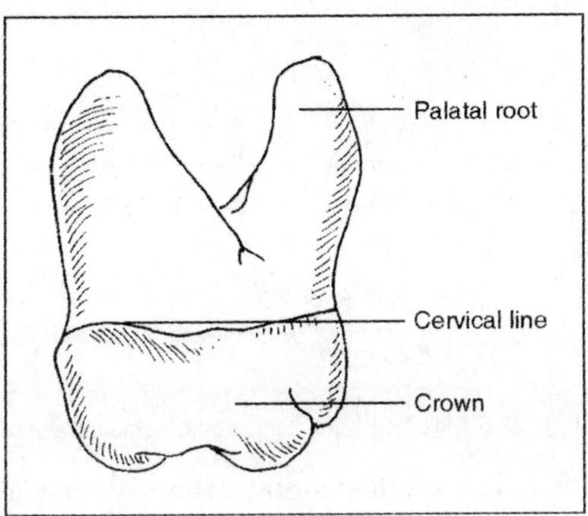

Fig. 22.3 Maxillary right first molar, mesial aspect

Distal aspect

Grossly the outline is similar to that of mesial aspect with little variation. Crown tapers distally hence most of buccal surface is visible from this aspect. Distal marginal ridge dips sharply in a cervical direction, exposing triangular ridges on distal portion cervical line is almost straight. Distobuccal root is narrower. Furcation lies more apical.

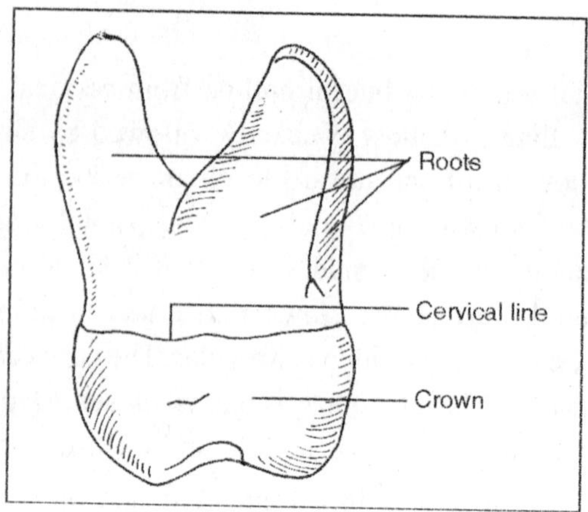

Fig. 22.4: Maxillary right first molar, distal aspect

Occlusal aspect

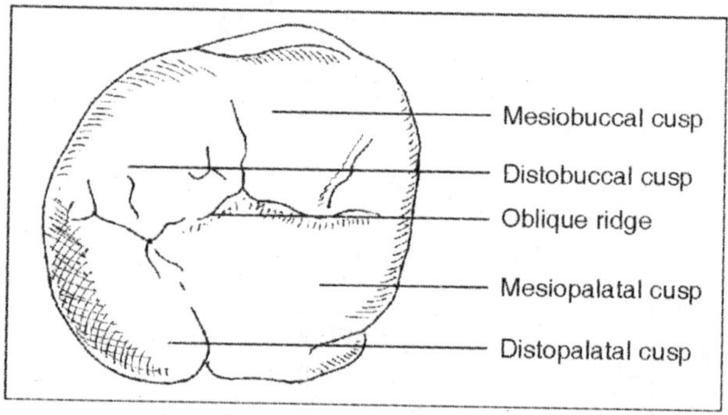

Fig. 22.5 Maxillary right fi.rst molar, occlusal aspect

Occlusally the maxillary 1st molors somewhat rhomboidal outlined by the four major cusp ridges and the marginal ridges. The four major cusps are well developed with the small minor or the fifth cusp appearing on mesiopalatal cusps. Mesiopalatal cusp in largest of all followed by MB, DL, DB and fifth cusp. There are two major fossae and two minor fossae. Central fossa which is triangular and mesial to obligue ridge and distal fossa roughly linear and distal to obligue ridge.

Two minor fossae are the mesial triangular fossa immediately distal to mesial marginal ridge and distal triangular fossa immediately mesial to distal marginal ridge.

Obligue ridge is a ridge that crosses the occlusal surface obliquelly that joins the triangular ridge of the distobuccal cusp and the distal ridge of he mesiolingual cusp.

L.Q.A.2 Write the difference between permanent maxillay 1st molar and permanent mandibular 1st molar

Ans. Difference between permanent maxillay 1st molar and permanent mandibular 1st molar.

Maxillary 1st molar	Mandibular 1st molar
• Eruption = 6 yrs	• 6 yrs but erupts earlier than maxillary first molar
• It is greater than the mandibular 1st molar	• Smaller as compaired to maxillary 1st molar
• It has well developed four cusps mesiobuccal mesiolingua, Distobuccal and Distopalatal and supplemental cusp Called cusp of cereblli	• It has well developed five cups mesiobuccal cusp, distobuccal cusp, distopalatal cusp, mesiolingual and small distal cusp.
• Palatal cusps of maxillary 1st molar are functional cusps.	• Buccal cusps of mandibular functional cusps.
• Cusp of carabelli is a supplemental cusp.	• It is not present on the mandibular 1st molar.
• Occusal surface rhomboidal	• Occlusal surface some what hexagonal
• Developmental grooves on occlusal surface, are Buccal groove, central groove, lingual groove distal, obligue groove, transvers groove and central pit.	• Develeopmental grooves central groove, MD groove, distobuccal groove, and lingual development grooves
• *Roots:* Maxillary 1st molar have 3 roots palatal, mesiobuccal & mesolingual	• *Roots:* It has two roots mesial and distal

S.A.Q.1 Cusp of carabelli (Tubercle of carabelli)

Ans. It is a supplemental cusp that is present on the mesiopalatal surface of the mesiopalatal cusp of maxillary 1st molar. It is a one of characteristic feature of maxillary 1st molar. It may be present as a well developed cusp/ tubercle or some time it is present as groove. It is outlined occlusally by an irregular developmental groove.

NOTES

23 Permanent Mandibular Molar

L.Q.A.1 Write briefly on occlusal aspect of mandibular permanent 2nd molar

Ans. Mandibular 2nd molar is smaller than the 1st molar. It supplement the 1st molar in function. It has four well developed cusps and two well developed roots.

Eruption: 11 to 13 yrs

Occlusal aspect

Mostly the occlusal surface of the mandibular second molar are rectangular, exhibits more curvature of the outline of the crown distally than mesially showing a semicircular outline to the distocclusal surface is comparison with a square outline mesially. It has four well developed cusps that are mesiobuccal, distobuccal, mesiolingual and distolingual. The small distal cusp that is present is 1st molar is absent in the 2nd molar. There is no distobuccal developmental groove. The buccal and lingual developmental grooves meet the central developmental groove at right angle at the central pit. These groove devide the occlusal surface into four equal parts. The fissuere pattern of 2nd molar resembles the 'Y'

L.Q.A.2 Describe morphology of mandibular permanent 1st molar

Ans. Mandibular 1st molar is the largest tooth in the mandibular arch.

It has five well developed cusp, two buccal cusp and two lingual and distal. Two well developed roots, one mesial and one distal which are broad buccalingually.

Buccal aspect

It is roughly trapezoidal with cervical and occlusal outline representing the uneven sides of trapezoid. From this aspect all the five cups are visible. The two buccal cusps and the buccal potion of the distal cusp in the foreground with the tips of the lingual cups in the background. The tips of the lingual cusps in the background. The lingual cusps may be seen because they are higher then the others. Two developmental groove appears on the others. Two developmental groove appears on the buccal surface these are mesiobuccal developmental groove and the distobuccal developmental groove. The mesiobuccal developmental groove acts as a line of demarcation between mesiobuccal lobe and the distobuccal lobe. The latter groove separates distobuccal to be from the distal lobe. The buccal cups are relatively flat. The MD cusp in widest mesiodistally. Cervical line in commonly regular in outline dipping apically toward the root bifurcation.

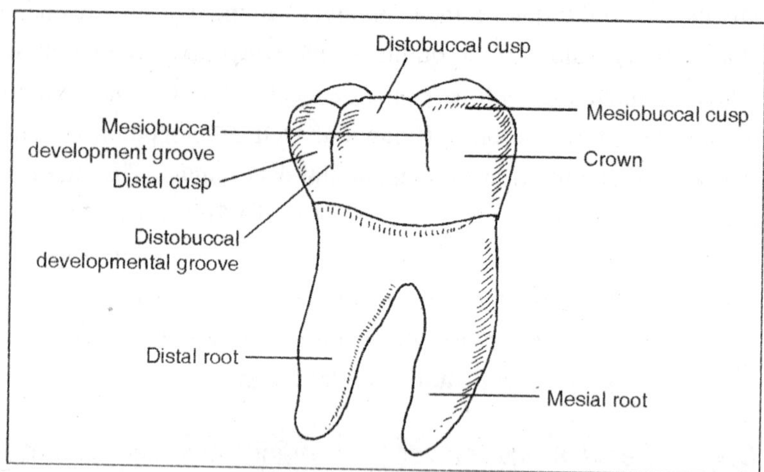

Fig. 23.1: Mandibular right first molar, buccal aspect

Both the roots are visible, mesial and distal. Mesial root is curved mesially from a point shortly below the cervical line to the middle 3rd position from which it curves distally. Distal root is less curved than mesial root and is also curved distally Apex of mesial root is blunt as compaired to distal root. Both roots are wider mesiodistally at the buccal areas than they are lingually.

Lingual aspect

From the lingual aspect three cusps are visible two lingual and lingual portion of distal cusps. As the lingual cusps are high enough they hide the buccal cusps. The mesiolingual cusp is widest mesiodistally and its tip is also highest that distolingual cusp. A developmental groove is present on thin surface which separates the mesiolingual and distolingual lobe called lingual developmental groove.

Mesial outline in convex from cervical line to marginal ridge distal outline is straight. Cervical line is irregular and tends to point sharply toward the root bifurcation. Root bifurcation at lingual aspect is 1 mm away as that of buccal surface.

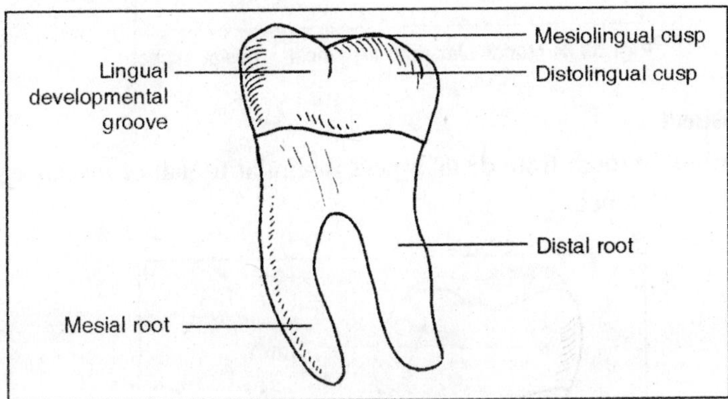

Fig. 24.2: Mandibular right first molar, lingual aspect

Mesial aspect

It appears roughly rhomboidal and the entire crown has a lingual tilt in relation to the root axis. When viewed mesially two cusps and one root is seen. Cusps visible are mesiobuccal and mesiolingual and the mesial surface of mesial root. Buccal outline is convex where as lingual outline is straight. The mesial marginal ridge is confluent with the mesial ridge of the mesiobuccal and mesiolingual cusps. Cervical line mesially is rather irregular and tends to curve occlusally about 1 mm toward centre of the mesial surface. Contact area is almost centered buccolingually in the mesial surface of the crown.

Mesial surface of mesial root is visible. Lingual outline is slanted in buccal direction although the outline is straight from cervical line. Buccal outline of mesial root drops straight down from the cervical line.

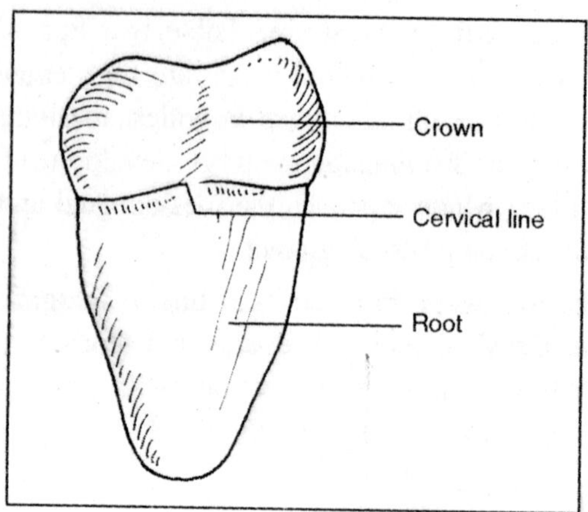

Fig. 23.3: Mandibular right first molar, mesial aspect

Distal aspect

Gross outline of tooth from distal aspect is similar to that of mesial aspect with little difference.

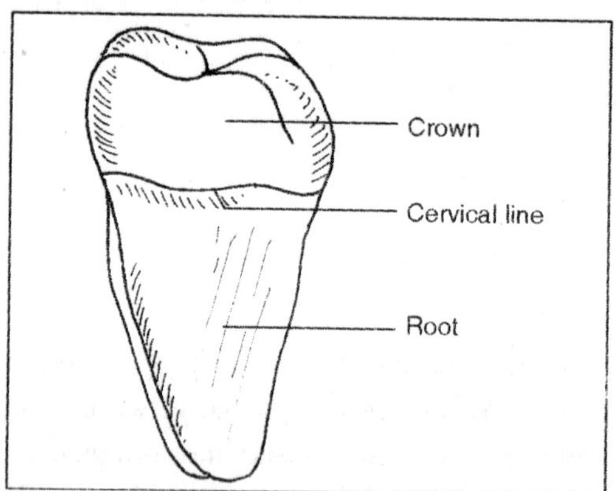

Fig. 23.4: Mandibular right first molar, distal aspect

Crown in shorter distally than mesially hence large part of tooth is visible and also because of distal convergence. Distal root is narrower buccalingually. Great part of occlusal surface is seen. Distal contact area is placed just below the distal cusp ridge of the distal cusp and at a slightly higher level above the cervical line than was found mesially. Distal marginal ridge is short and is made up of distal cusp ridge of distal cusp and the distolingual cusp ridge of distolingual cusp.

Cervical line is usually extends straight across buccolingually.

Occlusal aspect

Some what hexagonal outline. Development of cusp varies. Mesiobuccal cusp longer than either of two lingual cusps, which are equal to each other, the distobuccal cusp is smaller than any one of the above and the distal cusp is in most cases smallest of all.

Occlusal surface shows one major central fossa and two minor fossa these are mesial triangular fossa and distal triangular fossa.

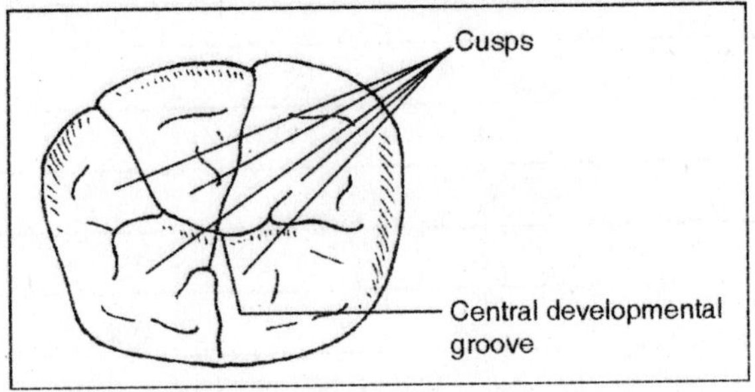

Fig. 23.5: Mandibular right first molar, occlusal aspect

Development grooves on occlusal surface are the central developmental groove, the mesiobuccal developmental groove, the distobuccal developmental groove and the lingual developmental groove.

NOTES

24

Dentoosseous Structure

L.Q.A.1 Describe blood & nerve supply of maxillary teeth

Ans.

Arterial supply

The arterial supply to the jaw bones and the teeth comes from the internal maxillary artery which is a branch of external carotid artery.

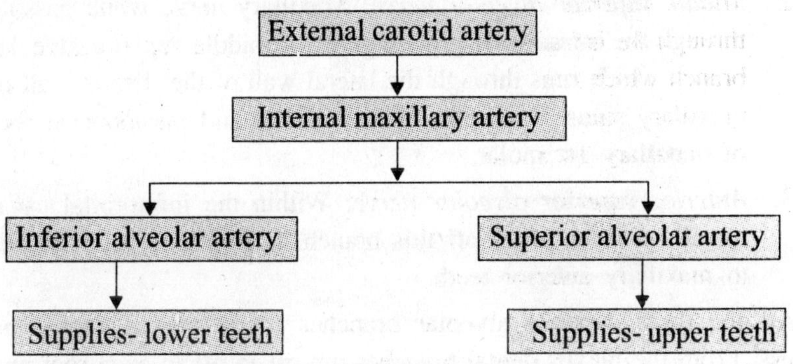

Arterial supply of maxillary teeth and jaw

Superior alveolar artery: It consist of three arteries.

1. *Posterior superior alveolar artery:* Branches from internal maxillary artery along with alveolar nerves, it supplies posterior teeth.
2. *Middle superior alveolar artery:* Branch given off by the intraorbital branch of internal maxillary artery. It runs downward

between the sinus mucosa and bone, ultimately supplies the maxillary teeth.

3. *Interior superior alveolar nerve:* Arises from the intra orbital artery before it emerges from foramen. It course down in anterior aspect of maxilla in bony canals to supply the maxillary teeth.

Nerve supply of maxillary teeth

It is through the maxillary nerve from its branches namely

- Posterior superior alveolar nerve
- Middle superior alveolar nerve
- Anterior superior alveolar nerve

1. *Posterior superior alveolar nerve:* Pterygopalatine portion of maxillary nerve gives this branch that enters the foramina present on the posterior surface of maxilla, forms plexus and supplies to the roots of maxillary molars except the mesiobuccal root of maxillary 1st molar.
2. *Middle superior alveolar nerve:* Maxillary nerve while passing through the infraorbital groove gives of middle superior alveolar branch which runs through the lateral wall of the lateral wall of maxillary sinus. It supplies the premolars and mesiobuccal root of maxillary 1st molar.
3. *Anterior superior alveolar nerve:* Within the infraorbital canal maxillary nerve gives off this branch. It distribute its, branches to maxillary anterior teeth.

All the three superior alveolar branches forms plexus above the process. From the plexus dental branches are given off to each root and interdental branches to bone, PDL and gingiva.

S.Q.A.1 Write briefly about lingual nerve

Ans. It is one of the two terminal branches of the posterior division of the mandibular nerve. It is sensory to the anterior 2/3 rd of the tongue and to the floor of the mouth.

Course and relationships

It begins just below the skull. Then it runs between the tensor palati and lateral pterygoid and then between lateral pterygoid and medial pterygoid.

About 2 cm. below the skull it is joined by the chordatympani nerve. After emerging from the lateral pterygoid the nerve runs downwards and forwards between the ramus and medial pterygoid. Next it lies in direct contact with the mandible medial to the 3rd molar. It than runs deep to the hyoglossous deep to the mylohyoid. Finally it lies on the surface of the genioglossus deep to the mylohyoid it winds oround the submandibular duct and divides into its terminal branches.

S.Q.A.2 Ramus of mandible

Ans. The mandible is the largest and strongest bone of the face. It has a horse shoe shaped body which lodges the teeth, a pair of rami which projects upward from the posterior end of the body and provide attachment to muscles.

Ramus

It is quadrilateral in shape and has two surfaces lateral and medial four borders upper, lower, presterior and anterior. Two process coronoid and condyloid process.

Lateral surface is flat and bears a number of oblique ridges.

Medial surface presents the following: Mandibular foreman, lingula, mylohyoid groove.

Upper border is thin and has notch called mandibular notch.

Muscle attachment

Temporalis: anterior border of coroid process *medial pterygoid:* on medial surface at angle region.

Sphenomandibular ligament: at lingula

lateral pterygoid: at pterygoid fovea

Massater: whole of lateral surface.

S.Q.A.3 Inferior dental nerve

Ans. It is the largest terminal branch of the posterior division of the mandibular nerve. It runs vertically downwards lateral to the medial pterygoid and to the sphenomandibular ligament. It enters the mandibular foramen and runs in the mandibular canal.

Branches

1. *Mylohyoid branch:* Contains all the motor fibers of the posterior division. It supplies the mylohyoid muscle and anterior belly of digastric
2. While passing through mandibular canal the inferior alveolar nerve branches that supply the lower teeth and gums.
3. The mental nerve is the terminal branch of inferior alveolar nerve that emerges from mental foramen and supplies the skin of the chin, mucous membrane etc. of lower lip.

NOTES

25 Occlusion

L.Q.A.1 Describe in detail about relationship of maxillary and mandibular permanent teeth

Ans. The facial and lingual relations of each tooth in one arch to its antagonist in the opposing arch is centric occlusion. In centric occlusion, facial views of the normal denture show each tooth of one arch in the opposing arch with the exception of the mandibular central incisors and the maxillary third molars. Each of the exceptions named has one antagonist only in the opposing jaw. Each tooth in one jaw will contact two teeth in the opposing jaw when in centric occlusion. An individual tooth, a posterior especially, will have most of its occlusal surface in contact with its namesake and adversary in the opposite jaw.

Since each tooth has two antagonists, the loss of one still leaves one antagoinst remaining, which will keep the tooth in occlusal contact with the opposing arch and keep it in its own arch relation at the same time by preventing elongation and displacement through the lack of antagonism. Actually, the loss of one or more teeth may precipitate a gradual disintegration of the occlusal relation of the dental arches unless a prosthetic replacement is made. The normal tooth arrangement minimizes the loss, however, and serves to resist immediate disintegration of the alignment.

The dental arches are composed throughout by teeth in pairs, starting at the median line, one right, one left, Each pair is made up of two teeth alike in form and dimension, but since one is right and the other left, The outline form is reversed from one side to the other to accommodate the situation. Central incisors only are in contact with each other at the median line; other pairs are divided distal to the centrals and each member of each pair will be to the left or to the right and will be in contact on both of its sides with other members of other pairs. Each arch is symmetrical bilaterally. The division into halves occurs at the median line. Both maxiallary and mandibular central incisors are in contact at this point, the only teeth in both arches with contact areas and embrasures directly in line with each other. All the other points of contact with associated embrasures, when located in one arch, are offset mesially or distally from contact and embrasure locations in the opposing arch. The contacts and embrasures of one arch are not equally measured from those in the opposing arch at any one location because of variations in the relative size of teeth.

The mandibular arch is narrower when calibrated at the buccal surfaces of posterior teeth than is the maxially arch. This relation is brought about by the differences the mesiodistal width between mandibular and maxillary anterior teeth (particularly the incisors) and by the lingual projection of mandibular posterior tooth crownsm, an arrangement that brings about proper intercuspation.

Horizontal overlap (overjet) is that characteristic of the teeth in which the incisal ridges or buccal cusp ridges of the maxillary teeth extend labially or buccally to the incisal ridges or buccal cusp ridges of the mandibular teeth, when the teeth are in centric occlusal relation.

Vertical overlap (overbite) is that characteristic of the teeth in which the incisal ridges of the maxillary anterior teeth extend below the incisal ridges of the mandibular anterior teeth when the teeth are placed in centric occlusal relation. Lingual views of the occlusal relations with the teeth in centric occlusion (Fig.) show the intercuspation of lingual cusp and how far the maxillary teeth occlude laterally to the lingual cusps of the mandibular arch.

The occlusal contact and intercusp relations of all the teeth of one arch with those in the opposing arch in centric occlusion:

Centric stops are areas of contact that a supporting cusp makes with opposing teeth. Thus the mesial lingual cusp of the maxillary first molar (a supporting cusp) makes contact with the central fossa (central stop) of the mandibular first molar. Centric occlusion is frequently the position of the jaw for bracing during swallowing and the terminal positon of the masticatory stroke.

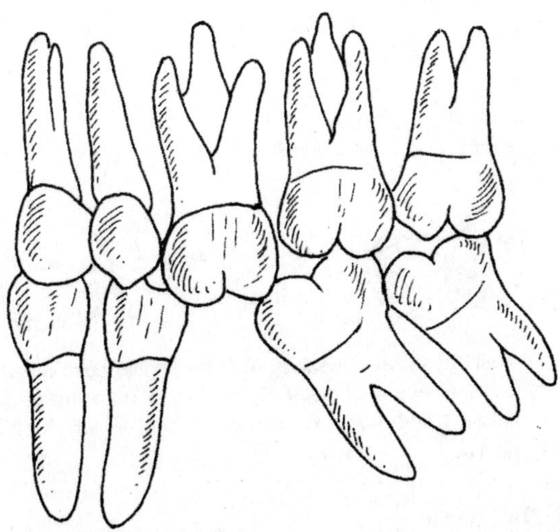

Fig. 25.1: This illustration demonstrates possible migration and improper contact and occlusal relation resulting from the loss of a mandibular first molar.

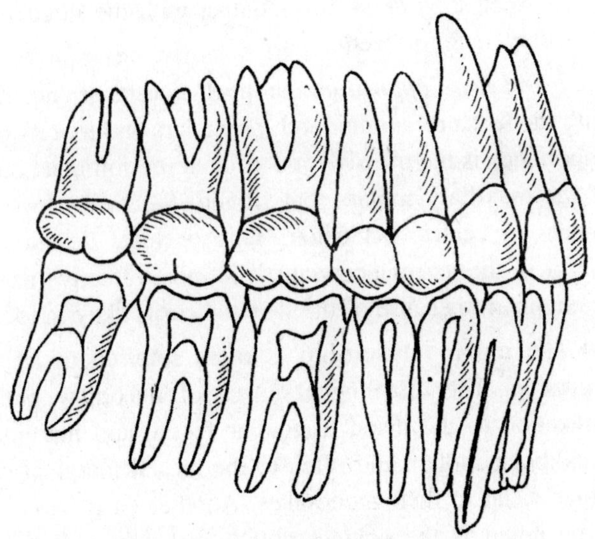

Fig. 25.2: Schematic drawing the facial relations of teeth in opposing arches in an idealized occlusion

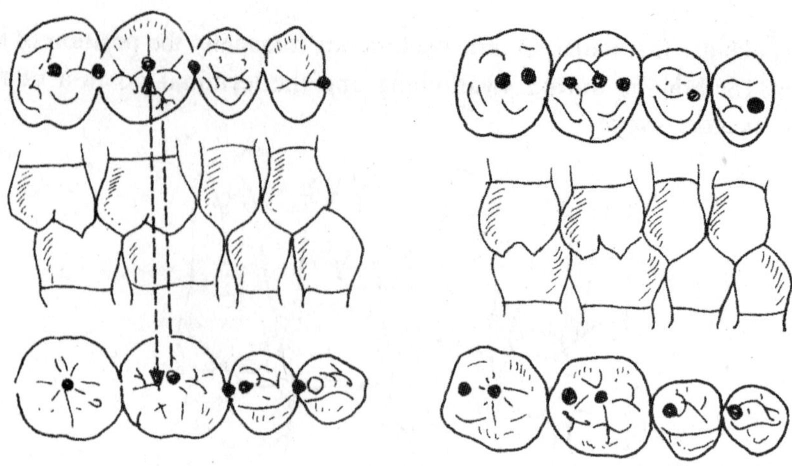

Fig. 25.3: Idealized cusp-fossa relationships. A, Mesiolingual cusp of maxillary first molar occluding in central fossa of lower first molar. Distal cusp of mandibular first molar occludes in central fossa of maxillary first molar. B, oclusal concept, in which all supporting cusps occlude in fossae.

Occlusion of the teeth

1. ***Surface contact:*** These contacting occlusal surfaces are found at incisal portions of mandibular anteriors, which becomes functional when they come into contact with the lingual surfaces of maxillary anterior teeth.
2. ***Cusp and fossa apposition:*** In this the cusps of one arch occludes with the fossa of another arch premolars and molars of particular importance is the massive and pointed mesiolingual cusp portions of the maxillary molars that fit into the major fossae of lower molars in centric occlusion. This occlusal design is not only useful in the act of chewing; it is most effective as a stabilizer of alignment because of the way the cusps "key in to" the fossae.

   The molar relationship is often referred to as the key to occlusion. The distolingual cusps of maxiallry molars are in apposition to the distal triangular fossae and marginal ridge of mandibular molars and often to the mesial marginal ridge of the molar distal to their namesakes. Another cusp-fossa relationship to be noted is the contact of relatively sharp lingual cusps of maxillary premolars with triangular-fossae of mandibular premolars.

The cusp-fossa apposition, including the buccal cusps of mandibular posterior teeth, follows:

The mesiobuccal cusps of mandibular molars are in apposition to the distal fossa, or the marginal ridge bordering it, of the tooth above, mesial to its namesake (e.g.1st molar mandibular to distal of 2nd maxillary premolar)

The buccal cusp tip of the second mandibular premolar approaches the mesial occlusal fossa of the opposing second premolar, while the first mandibular premolar occludes partly with the first premolar above and partly with the maxillary canine.

3. ***Cusp and embrassure apposition:*** Under this heading, some description is made that is often omitted when defining normal occlusion in centric occlusion. Some cusp tips are actually opposed to embrasure spaces. Other cusps are in partial contact with marginal and cusp ridges, in addition to stradding the embrasure spaces created by the ridges.
4. ***Ridge and sulcus apposition:*** Triangular ridges, a continuation of prominently formed enamel that extends from cusp tips toward the center of occlusal surfaces. The main ridge and sulcus oclusion that dominates discussion is that of the triangular ridges of the buccal cusps of maxillary molars as they are accommodated into buccal grooves with their sulci in mandibular molars. Another important combination is that of the triangular ridge of the distolingual cusp of the mandibular first molar as fits into the lingual groove sulcus of the maxillary first molar. Sulci are linear depressions between these enamel ridges with developmental grooves at the bottom of the enamel valleys.

S.Q.A.1 Overjet and overbite

Ans.

Overjet

Horizontal overlap is that characteristic of the teeth in which the incisal ridges or buccal cusp ridges of the maxillary extends labially or buccally to the incisal ridges of mandibular teeth normally it is 2 to 3 mms.

Overbite

Vertical overlap is that characteristic of the teeth in which the incisal ridges of the maxillary anterior teeth extends below the incisal ridges of mandibular anterior teeth. when the teeth are in centric relation. Normally 2 to 3 mms.

NOTES

NOTES

NOTES

NOTES

NOTES

NOTES

NOTES